李時珍先生原本

乾隆甲辰年冬

蘇郡總學張青萬仝校

張青萬重訂

書業堂

鐫藏

本草綱目

重訂本草綱目序

顧鄙老生既病且憚負

此二患世莫能醫其對

案不食憑牀不寐則病

之篤也醫書堆於前而

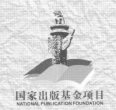

中华医药卫生

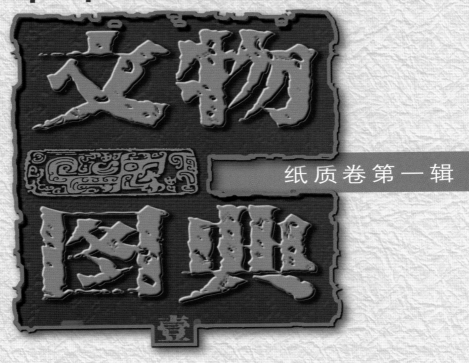

文物图典

纸质卷第一辑

主 编 李经纬 梁 峻 刘学春
总主译 白永权
主 译 吉 乐

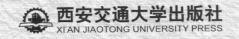

西安交通大学出版社
XI'AN JIAOTONG UNIVERSITY PRESS

图书在版编目 (CIP) 数据

中华医药卫生文物图典 . 1. 纸质卷 . 第 1 辑 . / 李经纬，
梁峻，刘学春主编 . — 西安：西安交通大学出版社，2016.12

ISBN 978-7-5605-7021-1

Ⅰ . ①中… Ⅱ . ①李… ②梁… ③刘… Ⅲ . ①中国医药学—
纸制品—文物—中国—图录 Ⅳ . ① R-092 ② K870.2

中国版本图书馆 CIP 数据核字（2015）第 022431 号

书　　名	中华医药卫生文物图典（一）纸质卷第一辑	
主　　编	李经纬　梁　峻　刘学春	
责任编辑	秦金霞	

出版发行　西安交通大学出版社

　　　　　（西安市兴庆南路 10 号　邮政编码 710049）

网　　址　http://www.xjtupress.com

电　　话　（029）82668805　82668502（医学分社）

　　　　　（029）82668315（总编办）

传　　真　（029）82668280

印　　刷　中煤地西安地图制印有限公司

开　　本　889mm×1194mm　1/16　　印张 30.25　字数 509 千字

版次印次　2017 年 12 月第 1 版　2017 年 12 月第 1 次印刷

书　　号　ISBN 978-7-5605-7021-1

定　　价　980.00 元

读者购书、书店添货、如发现印装质量问题，请通过以下方式联系、调换。

订购热线：（029）82665248　（029）82665249

投稿热线：（029）82668805　（029）82668502

读者信箱：medpress@126.com

铭记感受历史

自信自重自强

书贺

中华医药卫生文物图典问世

陈可冀 谨题

二〇一七年春日

陈可冀　中国科学院院士、国医大师

精修醫藥衛生文物
圖典功著當代
深究岐黄學術思想
渊源惠澤千秋
中華醫藥衛生文物圖典出版誌慶
丁酉孟秋 孫光榮 敬題於北京

孙光荣　国医大师

中華醫藥衛生文物圖典出版

彰顯中醫藥文化精神

體現中醫藥歷史價值

歲次丁酉夏　王琦

王琦　国医大师

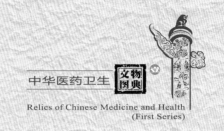

中华医药卫生

Relics of Chinese Medicine and Health
(First Series)

中华医药卫生文物图典（一）
丛书编撰委员会

主　编　李经纬　梁　峻　刘学春

副主编　廖　果　吴鸿洲　康兴军　和中浚　刘小斌　杨金生

　　　　　郑怀林　徐江雁　白建疆　黄　煌

编　委　李洪晓　梁永宣　王强虎　董树平　马　健　王　霞

　　　　　张雅宗　朱德明　包哈申　张建青　郑　蓉　庄乾竹

　　　　　李宏红　刘哲峰　王宏才　陈润东

总主译　白永权

主　译　陈向京　聂文信　范晓晖　温　睿　赵永生　杜彦龙

　　　　　吉　乐　李小棉　郭　梦　陈　曦

副主译（按姓氏音序排列）

　　　　　董艳云　姜雨孜　李建西　刘　慧　马　健　任宝磊

　　　　　任　萌　任　莹　王　颇　习通源　谢皖吉　徐素云

　　　　　许崇钰　许　梅　詹菊红　赵　菲　邹郝晶

译 者（按姓氏音序排列）

迟征宇　邓　甜　付一豪　高　琛　高　媛　郭　宁

韩　蕾　何宗昌　胡勇强　黄　鋆　蒋新蕾　康晓薇

李静波　刘雅恬　刘妍萌　鲁显生　马　月　牛笑语

唐云鹏　唐臻娜　田　多　铁红玲　佟健一　王　晨

王　丹　王　栋　王　丽　王　媛　王慧敏　王梦杰

王仙先　吴耀均　席　慧　肖国强　许子洋　闫红贤

杨姣姣　姚　晔　张　阳　张　鋆　张继飞　张梦原

张晓谦　赵　欣　赵亚力　郑　青　郑艳华　朱江嵩

朱瑛培

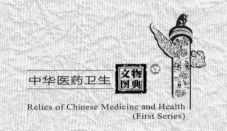

中华医药卫生
Relics of Chinese Medicine and Health
(First Series)

本册编撰委员会

丛书策划委员会

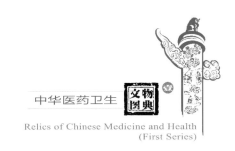

中华医药卫生 文物图典

Relics of Chinese Medicine and Health
(First Series)

序 言

　　探索天、地、人运动变化规律以及"气化物生"过程的相互关系，是人类永恒的课题。宇宙不可逆，地球不可逆，人生不可逆业已成为共识。天地造化形成自然，人类活动构成文化。文物既是文化的载体，又是物化的历史，还是文明的见证。

　　追求健康长寿是人类共同的夙愿。中华民族之所以繁衍昌盛，健康文化起了巨大的推动作用。由于古人谋求生存发展、应对环境变化产生的智慧，大多反映在以医药卫生为核心的健康文化之中，所以，习总书记说："中医药学是中国古代科学的瑰宝，也是打开中华文明宝库的钥匙"。

　　秉持文化大发展、大繁荣理念，中国中医科学院李经纬、梁峻等为负责人的科研团队在完成科技部"国家重点医药卫生文物收集调研和保护"课题获 2005 年度中华中医药学会科技二等奖基础上，又资鉴"夏商周断代工程""中华文明探源工程"等相关考古成果，用有重要价值的新出土文物置换原拍摄质量较差的文物，适当补充民族医药文物，共精选收载 5000 余件。经西安交通大学出版社申报，《中华医药卫生文物图典（一）》（以下简称《图典》）于 2013 年获得了国家出版基金的资助，并经专业翻译团队翻译，使《图典》得以面世。

　　文物承载的信息多元丰富，发掘解读其中蕴藏的智慧并非易事。医药卫生文物更具有特殊性，除文物的一般属性外，还承载着传统医学发展史迹与促进健康的信息。运用历史唯物主义观察发掘文物信息，善于从生活文物中领悟卫生信息，才能准确解读其功能，也才能诠释其在民生健康中的历史作用，收到以古鉴今之效果。"历史是现实的根源"，任何一个民族都不能割断历史，史料都包含在文化中。"文化是民族的血脉，是人民的精神家园"，文化繁荣才能实现中华民族的伟大复兴。值本《图典》付梓之际，用"梳理文化之脉，必获健康之果"作为序言并和作者、读者共勉！

中央文史研究馆馆员
中国工程院院士　王永炎
丁酉年仲夏

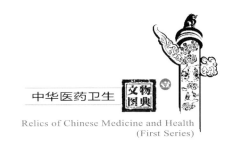

前 言

　　文化是相对自然的概念，是考古界常用词汇。文物是文化的重要组成部分，既是文明的物证，又是物化的历史。狭义医药卫生文物是疾病防治模式语境下的解读，而广义医药卫生文物则是躯体、心态、环境适应三维健康模式下的诠释。中华民族是56个民族组成的多元一体大家庭，中华医药卫生文物当然包括各民族的健康文化遗存。

　　天地造化如造山、板块漂移、气候变迁、生物起源进化等形成自然。气化物生莫贵于人，即整个生物进化的最高成果是人类自身。广义而言，人类生存思维留下的痕迹即物质财富和精神财富总和构成文化，其一般的物化形式是视觉感知的文物、文献、胜迹等。其中质变标志明晰的文化如文字、文物、城市、礼仪等可称作文明。从唯物史观视角观察，狭义文化即精神财富，尤其体现人类精、气、神状态的事项，其本质也具有特殊物质属性，如量子也具有波粒二相性，这种粒子也是物质，无非运动方式特殊而已。现代所谓可重复验证的"科学"，事实上也是从文化中分离出来的事项，因此也是一种特殊文化形式。追求健康长寿是人类共同的夙愿。中华民族之所以繁衍昌盛，是因为健康文化异彩纷呈。中华优秀传统医药文化之所以博大精深，是因为其原创思维博大、格物致知精深，所以，习总书记说："中医药学是中国古代科学的瑰宝，也是打开中华文明宝库的钥匙"。

文化既反映时代、地域、民族分布、生产资料来源、技术水平等信息，又反映人类认知水平和生存智慧。发掘解读文物、文献中蕴藏的健康知识和灵动智慧，首先是从事健康工作者的责任和义务。《易经》设有"观"卦，人类作为观察者，不仅要积极收藏展陈文物，而且要善于捕捉文物倾诉的信息，汲取养分，启迪思维，收到古为今用之效果。墨子三表法，首先一表即"本之于古者圣王之事"，也是强调古代史实的重要性。"历史是现实的根源"，现实是未来的基础。任何一个国家、地区、民族都不能割断历史、忽略基础，这个基础就是文化。"文化是民族的血脉，是人民的精神家园"。文化繁荣才能驱动各项事业发展，才能实现中华民族的伟大复兴。

人类从类人猿分化出来。"禄丰古猿禄丰种"是云南禄丰发现的类人猿化石，距今七八百万年。距今 200 万年前人类进入旧石器时代，直立行走，打制石器产生工具意识，管理火种，是所谓"燧人氏"时代。中国留存有更新世早、中期的元谋、蓝田、北京人等遗址。距今 10 万—5 万年前，人类进入旧石器时代中期，即早期智人阶段，脑容量增加，和欧洲、非洲人种相比，原始蒙古人种颧骨前突等，是所谓"伏羲氏"时代。中国发现的马坝、长阳、丁村人等较典型。距今 5 万—1 万年前，人类进入旧石器时代晚期，即晚期智人阶段，细石器、骨角器等遍布全国，山顶洞、柳江、资阳人等较典型。

中石器时代距今约 1 万年，是旧石器时代向新石器时代的短暂过渡期，弓箭发明，狗被驯化。河南灵井、陕西沙苑遗址等作为代表。距今 1 万—公元前 2600 年前后，人类进入新石器时代，磨光石器、烧制陶器，出现农业村落并饲养家畜，是所谓"神农氏"时代。公元前 7000 年以来，在甲、骨、陶、石等载体上出现契刻符号、七音阶骨笛乐器等，反映出人文气息趋浓。公元前 6000—公元前 3500 年的老官台、裴李岗、河姆渡、马家浜、仰韶等文化遗址，彰显出先民围绕生存健康问题所做的各种努力。

公元前 4800 年以来，以关中、晋南、豫西为中心形成的仰韶文化，是中原史前文化的重要标志。以半坡、庙底沟类型为典型，自公元前 3500 年走向繁荣，属于锄耕粟黍稻兼营渔猎饲养猪鸡经济方式，彩陶尤其发达。公元前 4400—公元前 3300 年，长江中游的大溪文化，薄胎彩陶和白陶发达。公元前 4300—公元前 2500 年山东丰岛的大汶口文化，红陶为主。公元前 3500 年前后，辽东的红山文化原始宗教发展。公元前 3300 年以来，长江下游由河姆渡、马家浜文化衍续的良渚文化和陇西的马家窑文化、江淮间的薛家岗文化时趋发达。

公元前 2600—公元前 2000 年，黄河中下游龙山文化群形成，冶铸铜器，制作玉器，土坯、石灰、夯筑技术开始应用。公元前 2697 年，轩辕战败炎帝（有说其后裔）、蚩尤而为黄帝纪元元年。黄帝西巡访贤，"至岐见岐伯，引载而归，访于治道"。其引归地"溱洧襟带于前，梅泰环拱于后"，即今河南新密市古城寨。岐黄答问，构建《黄帝内经》健康知识体系，中华文明从关注民生健康起步。颛顼改革宗教，神职人员出现；帝喾修身节用，帝尧和合百国，舜同律度量衡，大禹疏导治水，中华民族不断繁衍昌盛。

公元前 2070 年，禹之子启以豫西晋南为中心建立夏王朝，二里头青铜文化为其特征，半地穴、窑洞、地面建筑并存。饮食卫生器具、酒器增多。朱砂安神作用在宫殿应用。公元前 1600 年，商灭夏。偃师商城设有铸铜作坊。公元前 1300 年，盘庚迁殷，使用甲骨文。武丁时期青铜浑铸、分铸并存。公元前 1056 年，相传周"文王被殷纣拘于羑里，演《周易》，成六十四卦"。公元前 1046 年，武王克商建周，定都镐京。青铜器始铸长篇铭文，周原发掘出微型甲骨文字。公元前 770 年，平王东迁。虢国铸铜柄铁剑。公元前 753 年，秦国设置史官。公元前 707 年出现蝗灾、公元前 613 年出现"哈雷彗星"，均被孔子载入《春秋》。公元前 221 年，秦始皇统一中国，多元一体民族大家庭形成，中华医药卫生文物异彩纷呈。

中国是治史大国，历来重视发展文化博物事业，1955 年成立卫生部中医研究院时就设置医史研究室，1982 年中国医史文献研究所成立时复建中国医史博物馆研究收藏展陈文物。2000—2003 年，经王永炎院士、姚乃礼院长等呼吁，科技部批准立项，由李经纬、梁峻为负责人的团队完成"国家重点医药卫生文物收集调研和保护"项目任务，受到科技部项目验收组专家的高度评价，获中华中医药学会科技进步二等奖。2013 年，在国家出版基金资助下，课题组对部分文物重新拍摄或必要置换、充实民族医药文物后，由西安交通大学出版社编辑、组聘国内一流翻译团队英译说明文字付梓，受到国家中医药博物馆筹备工作领导小组和办公室的高度重视。

"物以类聚"，《图典》主要依据文物质地、种类分为 9 卷，计有陶瓷，金属，纸质，竹木，玉石、织品及标本，壁画石刻及遗址，少数民族文物，其他，备考等卷。同卷下主要根据历史年代或小类分册设章。每卷下的历史时段不求统一。遵循上述规则将《图典》划分为21册，总计收载文物5000余件。对每件文物的描述，除质地、规格、馆藏等基本要素外，重点描述其在民生健康中的作用。对少数暂不明确的事项在括号中注明待考。对引自各博物馆的材料除在文物后列出馆藏外，还在书后再次统一列出馆名或参考书目，以充分尊重其馆藏权，也同时维护本典作者的引用权。

21世纪，围绕人类健康的生命科学将飞速发展，但科学离不开文化，文化离不开文物。发掘文物承载的信息为现实服务，谨引用横渠先生四言之两语："为天地立心，为生民立命"，既作为编撰本《图典》之宗旨，也是我们践行国家"一带一路"倡议的具体努力。希冀通过本《图典》的出版发行，教育国人，提振中华民族精神；走向世界，为人类健康事业贡献力量。

李经纬　梁峻　刘学春

2017年6月于北京

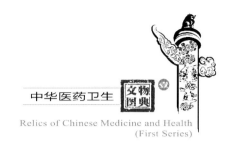

中华医药卫生 文物图典

Relics of Chinese Medicine and Health
(First Series)

目 录

第四章 清代（1840年以前）

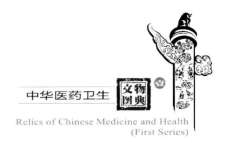

中华医药卫生 文物图典

Relics of Chinese Medicine and Health
(First Series)

Contents

Chapter Four Qing Dynasty(Before 1840)

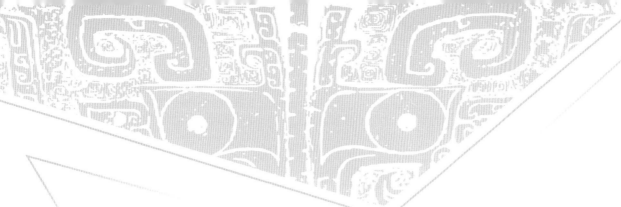

◈ 第一章　周至唐代

Chapter One　Zhou Dynasty to Tang Dynasty

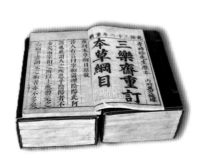

《周易参同契》书影

东汉

选自《神异典》第 293 卷之《静功部》，作者魏伯阳。文中对行气养生的方法、体系作了阐述，并以《周易》阴阳运动原理为骨架，以"黄老"精气学说为内核，借用丹鼎炉火等术语，构筑了行气练养术的理论模式。

中国国家图书馆藏

Book Photograph of *Zhou Yi Can Tong Qi*

Eastern Han Dynasty

The book was selected from *Jing Gong Bu*, the 293rd volume of *Shen Yi Dian*, an ancient book about health maintenance, written by Wei Boyang. The book elucidated the method and system of maintaining good health with Qi and constructed a theoretical model of "Xing Qi Lian Yang Shu" by taking the principle of movement of Yin and Yang in *Zhou Yi* (The Book of Changes) as the framework, "Huang Lao Essence Theory" as the core, and also borrowing some terminologies such as Dan (pill), Ding (tripod vessel), Lu (stove) and Huo (fire).

Preserved in National Library of China

手抄本《呼吸静功妙诀》

唐

《呼吸静功妙诀》于 1900 年在莫高窟藏经洞发现后被法国人伯希和劫走，编号为 P.3810。其正文凡 13 行，273 字，从字迹和抄写的水平上看，应为唐代道人的手抄本。它从行气养生的角度，以道家的观点，对通过"呼吸"的锻炼，进而达到提高生命境界和质量、延伸生命长度之目的作了细致的阐述，在养生学上具有重要意义。

法国国家图书馆藏

Manuscript of *Hu Xi Jing Gong Miao Jue* (Key to Use Breath)

Tang Dynasty

Hu Xi Jing Gong Miao Jue was discovered in the Sutra Cave of Dunhuang Mogao Grottoes in 1900. After its discovery, it was robbed by Frenchman Paul Pelliot. The serial number of *Hu Xi Jing Gong Miao Jue* is P. 3810. There are 13 lines and 273 characters. According to the style and level of its handwriting, it is believed to be the manuscript of a Taoist in the Tang Dynasty. In respect of the theory of Taoism, this book elaborates longevity through breath exercise to improve the level and quality of life. It plays an important role in the subject of health preservation.

Preserved in French National Library

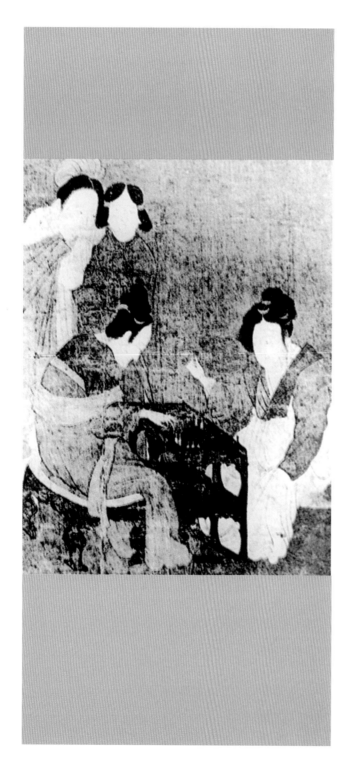

张萱《捣练图》局部

唐

原画已散失，此为宋徽宗赵佶临摹本。这里选取的是描绘唐代仕女打双陆的画面，图中双陆局为双层构架，每层开同样的壶门洞。捣衣捶状的黑白双陆子错落地摆在盘上。两个仕女正在聚精会神地对局，另一位则由侍女搀扶着站在旁边观看。

美国波士顿美术馆藏

Dao Lian Tu by Zhang Xuan (Partial)

Tang Dynasty

The original painting has been missing. This one was a copy painted by Zhao Ji, who was an emperor in the Song Dynasty. The excerpted part shows two ladies playing a game called Shuanglu. There are holes on both layers of the game table, on which black and white pieces scatter here and there. Two ladies are playing the game attentively. Another lady is watching while standing aside with her maid.

Preserved in Museum of Fine Arts, Boston

◇ 第二章 辽宋金元

Chapter Two　Liao, Song, Jin, and Yuan Dynasties

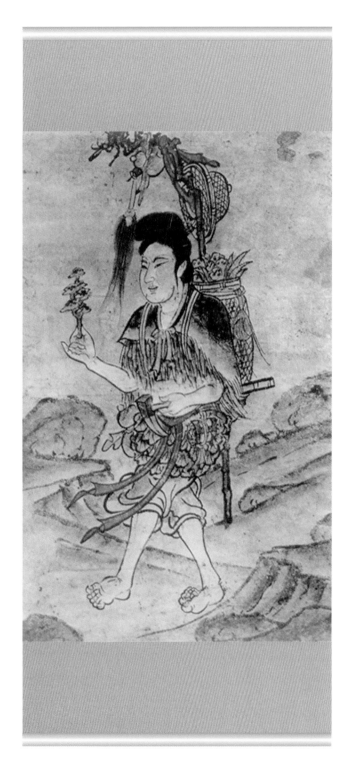

神农采药图

辽

纵 54 厘米，横 34.6 厘米

图中人物面部丰满，赤足袒腹，披兽皮，围叶裳，负竹篓，举灵芝，行于山石间。有研究者认为此乃神农。1974 年于山西应县佛宫寺木塔内发现。

山西博物院藏

Painting of Shennong Gathering Medical Plants

Liao Dynasty

Vertical Length 54 cm / Horizontal Length 34.6 cm

The figure in the painting has plumped cheeks and no covering on his feet and belly, taking animal skins as his clothes. He is walking in the hills with leaves around his waist, carrying a bamboo basket and holding a Ganoderma. Researchers think this figure is Shennong, the inventor of Chinese farming and medicine. It was discovered inside the Fogong Temple Pagoda in Yingxian County, Shanxi Province, in 1974.

Preserved in Shanxi Museum

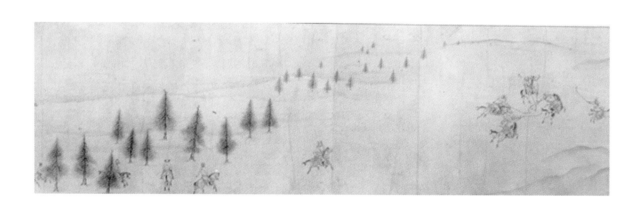

陈及之《便桥会盟图》卷局部

辽

原画：纵 36 厘米，横 77.4 厘米

墨笔。此图以唐太宗李世民（627—649 年在位）和突厥可汗颉利，在武德九年（626）于长安城西渭水便桥会盟之事实为背景绘制而成。这里选取的是这一长卷中唐、辽两国进行马球比赛画面的局部。画中数名骑士策马持杖在争击一球，场面热烈、壮观。

故宫博物院藏

Bian Qiao Hui Meng Tu by Chen Jizhi (Partial)

Liao Dynasty

Total Scroll: Vertical Length 36 cm/ Horizontal Length 77.4 cm

Its historical background is the alliance meeting between Li Shimin (famous emperor from 627 to 649 in the Tang Dynasty) and Ji Li (Khan of Tujue) at Weishui bridge in Chang'an City in 626. The excerpted part depicts the polo match between Tang and Liao. In this picture, several knights are batting a ball, which is very spectacular.

Preserved in The Palace Museum

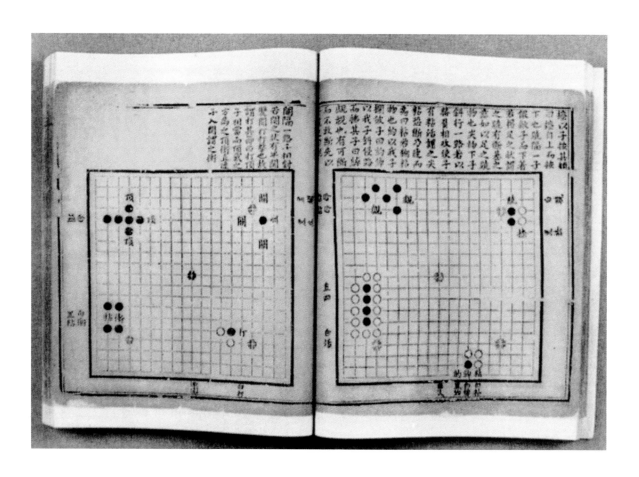

张凝《棋经十三篇》书影

北宋

竹纸

宽 32.4 厘米，高 27.8 厘米

《棋经十三篇》为北宋仁宗翰林学士张凝撰，明刊本，金镶玉线装。其内容包括论局、得算、权舆、合战、虚实、自知、审局、度情、斜正、洞微、名数、品格和杂说十三篇，对宋以前的围棋理论特别是战术原则作了详尽的论述，是我国古代流传下来的较早的围棋著作。

中国书店藏

Book Photograph of *Qi Jing Shi San Pian* by Zhang Ning

Northern Song Dynasty

Bamboo Paper

Width 32.4 cm / Height 27.8 cm

Qi Jing Shi San Pian, sewn with gold and jade, was compiled by Zhang Ning, an academician and official in the Northern Song Dynasty. The preserved one was the edition of the Ming Dynasty. This book includes 13 articles, discussing the theories and tactics principles of Weiqi before the Song Dynasty. It is a great work of Weiqi from early ages in China.

Preserved in China Bookshop

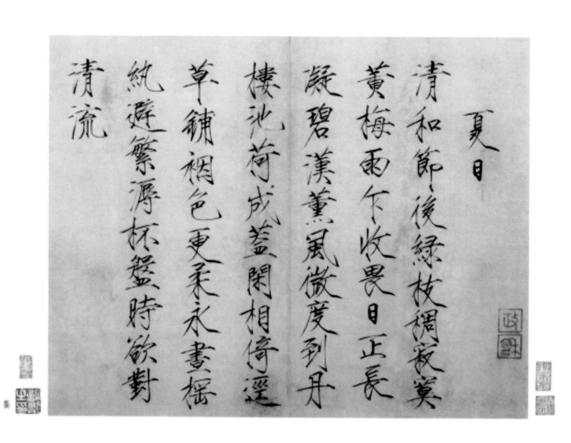

赵佶《夏日诗》帖

宋

纵 33.7 厘米，横 44.2 厘米

书法劲健舒展，为赵佶晚年之作。

故宫博物院藏

Xia Ri Shi (Poem of Summer) by Zhao Ji

Song Dynasty

Vertical Length 33.7 cm / Horizontal Length 44.2 cm

The calligraph is vigorous and forceful. It was written by Zhao Ji in his old age.

Preserved in The Palace Museum

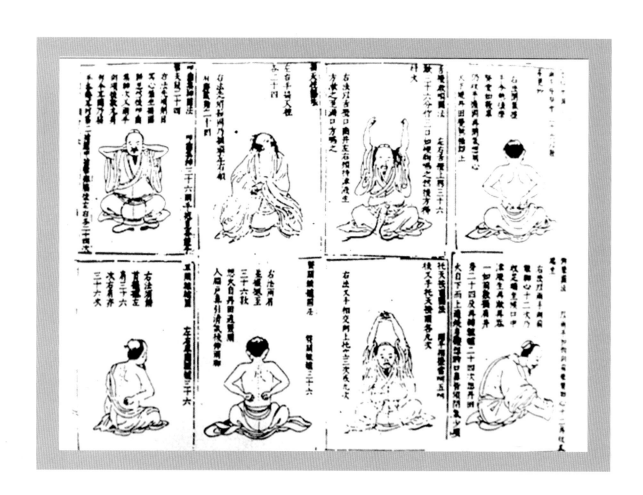

《文八段锦图谱》

南宋

该图谱创编于南宋初年，作者不详。八段锦凡八图，皆附文字说明，是一套由摇天柱、舌搅漱咽、摩肾堂、单关辘轳、双关辘轳、托天按项、钩攀等八节动作编排而成的导引式式。这里选取的是由中国国家图书馆所藏，明万历三十七年（1609）刊行的《三才图会》"人事"卷十所收录的《文八段锦图谱》。

中国国家图书馆藏

Wen Ba Duan Jin Tu Pu

Southern Song Dynasty

Wen Ba Duan Jin Tu Pu (Atlas of Chinese Traditional Medical Gymnastics in Sedentary Positions) was created by an unknown author in the early Southern Song Dynasty. Containing eight pictures with explanatory notes, it is a guiding exercise arranged by eight movements. The preserved one is from the 10th chapter of "Human Sector" in *San Cai Tu Hui* (an illustrated ancient Chinese encyclopedia about everything in the sky, the earth and the human world) published in 1609 during the reign of Emperor Wanli of the Ming Dynasty.

Preserved in National Library of China

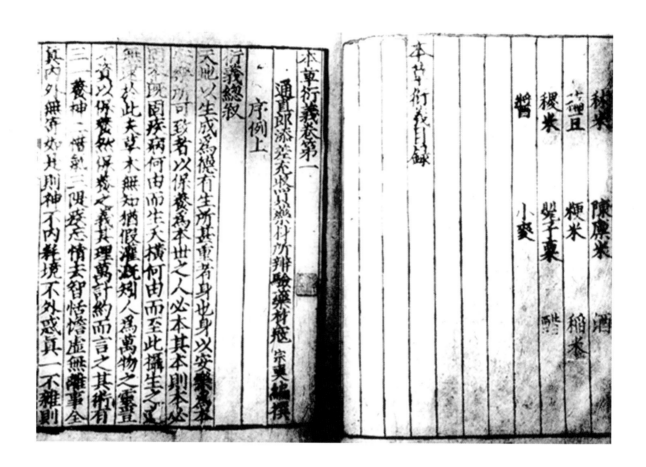

《本草衍义》书影

宋

宋刻本。寇宗奭撰。20卷。约成书于政和六年（1116）。本书为补充发挥《嘉祐补注本草》和《本草图经》二书未尽之意而著，故名。书中将《嘉祐补注本草》中有待深入探讨的药物约470种做了进一步的辨析和讨论，并有本草理论方面的论述。

首都图书馆藏

Book Photograph of *Ben Cao Yan Yi* (Expanded Herbal Foundation)

Song Dynasty

As the block-printed edition in the Song Dynasty, this book was written by Kou Zongshi in about 1116. Containing 20 chapters, this book was aimed at supplementing the two books named *Jia You Bu Zhu Ben Cao* and *Ben Cao Tu Jing*. And that is how it was named. This book further explored into 470 Chinese herbal medicines that were not fully discussed in *Jia You Bu Zhu Ben Cao*, as well as the theory of Chinese herbal medicine.

Preserved in Capital Library of China

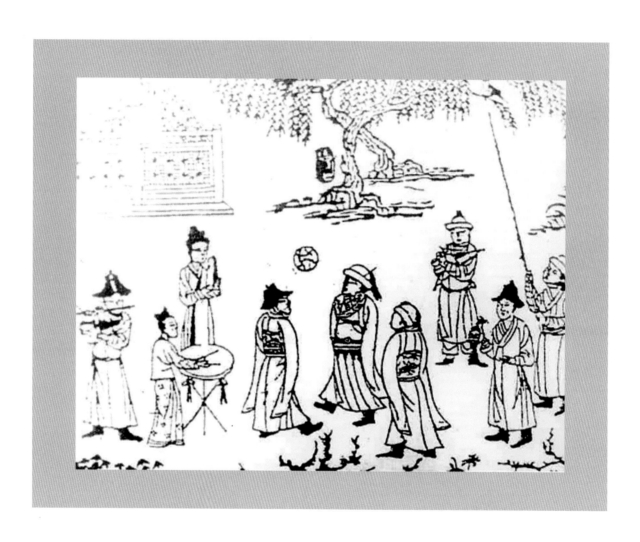

《事林广记·园社摸场图》

宋

《事林广记》42 卷，12 册，宋人陈元靓编著。元至顺年间（1330—1332）建安椿庄书院刻本。园杜摸场图载于《戍集》卷之七中，图中在鼓乐伴奏下，三人正进行"白打"式蹴鞠活动比赛。

中国国家图书馆藏

Shi Lin Guang Ji-Yuan She Mo Chang Tu

Song Dynasty

This painting is from *Shi Lin Guang Ji* (an encyclopedia-like book), which consists of 42 chapters and 12 volumes. This book was compiled by Chen Yuanjing in the Song Dynasty and was the block-printed edition by Jian'an Chunzhuang Academy during the Yuan Dynasty (1330–1332). This painting is among the 7th collection of *Shu Ji*, one of the chapters. In the picture, three men are playing Cuju (a kind of football game), accompanied by drum music.

Preserved in National Library of China

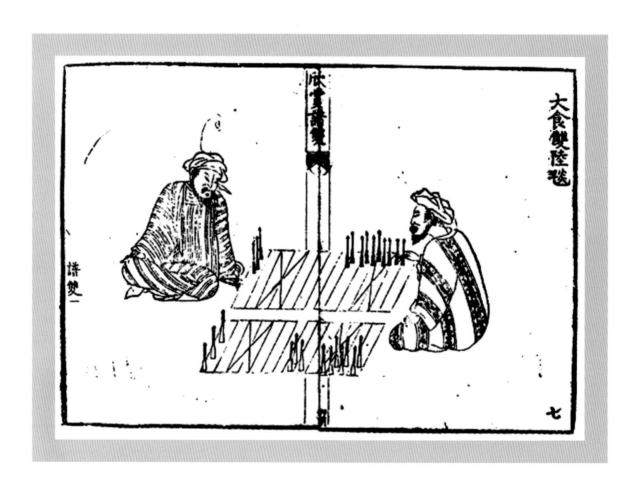

《谱双·大食双陆毯》

宋

框：纵 12.4 厘米，横 16.2 厘米

《谱双》，明万历年间（1573—1620）茅一相刊《欣赏编》本。宋代洪遵编著，此插图名为"大食双陆毯"，描绘了大食国（阿拉伯帝国）人打双陆的情景。

辽宁省博物馆藏

Pu Shuang- Da Yi Shuang Lu Tan

Song Dynasty

Frame: Vertical Length 12.4 cm/ Horizontal Length 16.2 cm

Pu Shuang (a book on skills and principles of backgammon) was compiled by Hong Zun and published by Mao Yixiang as an edition of *Xin Shang Bian* (a book about cultural recreational activities) during the reign of Emperor Wanli of the Ming Dynasty (1573–1620). This inset, called "Da Yi Shuang Lu Tan", describes a scene of Arabians playing backgammon.

Preserved in Liaoning Provincial Museum

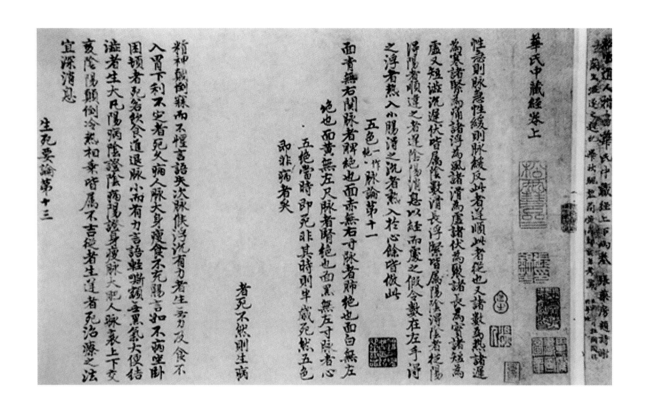

赵子昂书《中藏经》真迹（局部）

元

《中藏经》系综合性医书，旧题汉朝华佗撰，撰年不详（约成书于宋）。3卷。本书医论部分计49篇，论述脏腑生成、病机及辨证。后面部分介绍各科治疗方剂及其主治病症。本书作者经验丰富，所论颇有实用价值，故本书流传亦广。现有《医统正脉》等刊本。赵孟頫（1254—1322），字子昂，元代著名书画家。

上海博物馆藏

Authentic Work of *Central Treasury Canon* By Zhao Zi'ang (Partial)

Yuan Dynasty

Central Treasury Canon is a comprehensive medical book. It was written by Hua Tuo in the Han Dynasty, with unknown specific date (The book was completed approximately in the Song Dynasty). There are 3 chapters. In the medical sector, there are 49 articles discussing viscera growth, pathogenesis, and analysis. Another sector introduces treatment prescriptions and their indications. The rich experience of the author and the practical value of the analysis made the book broadly circulated. Now, there are editions like *Yi Tong Zheng Mai* and so on. Zhao Mengfu (1254–1322), courtesy name Zi'ang, was a famous calligrapher and painter in the Yuan Dynasty.

Preserved in Shanghai Museum

《千金要方》书影

元

元刻本。孙思邈约撰于公元652年。30卷。孙氏以"人命至重，有贵千金，一方济之，德逾于此"，故名。本书包括医学伦理、本草、临证各科等内容，计233门，合方5000余首。书中所载内容系统地总结和反映了自《黄帝内经》后至唐初中国医药学的发展，具有较高的学术价值，对国内外均有较为深远的影响。

中国中医科学院图书馆藏

Book Photograph of *Qian Jin Yao Fang* (Invaluable Prescriptions for Ready Reference)

Yuan Dynasty

The original book is the block-printed edition. The book was written by Sun Simiao in the year 652. There are 30 chapters. The name means that human life is as invaluable as gold and it would be great virtues to save a life with one prescription. This book includes medical theories, herbalism, and indications, with 233 categories and more than 5,000 prescriptions. This book systematically summaries and reflects the development of traditional Chinese medicine and pharmacy since the accomplishment of *Huang Di Nei Jing* (Inner Canon of the Yellow Emperor) till the early Tang Dynasty. It is a work with high academic value and exerts profound domestic and international influences. Preserved in Library of China Academy of Chinese Medical Sciences

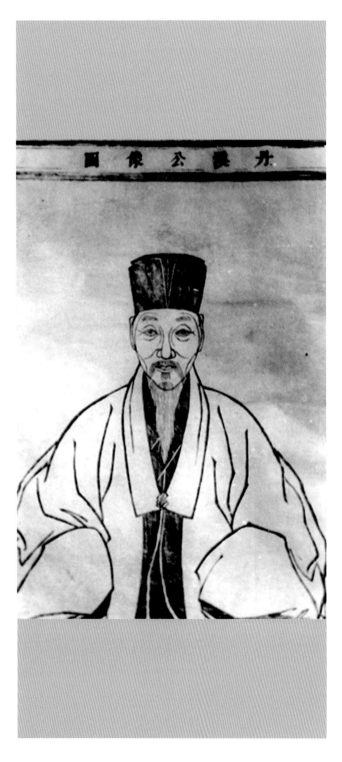

朱丹溪木刻像

元

朱震亨（1281—1358），字彦修，世称丹溪翁，婺州义乌（今浙江省义乌）人。初事许谦求道德性命之学，又从罗知悌学医，得刘完素、张从正、李杲之真传，阐发相火之根源，倡"阳常有余，阴常不足"论，治病颇验，冠称一时。著有《局方发挥》《格致余论》《脉因证治》等书。此像采自朱氏族谱。

浙江义乌冯汉龙藏

Wood Carving Statue of Zhu Danxi

Yuan Dynasty

Zhu Zhenheng(1281–1358), courtesy name Yanxiu, was also called Danxiweng. He was from Yiwu, Wuzhou (now in Zhejiang Province). He initially learned theory of morality and life from Xu Qian and then learned medicine from Luo Zhiti. He also received the core theories of Liu Wansu, Zhang Congzheng, and Li Gao. He elucidated the theory of essence of life and advocated a theory that sickness mostly resulted from the excessive Yangqi and insufficient Yinqi, which was highly efficacious and made him famous at that time. He also wrote other books like *Ju Fang Fa Hui, Ge Zhi Yu Lun, Mai Yin Zheng Zhi* and so on. This statue was copied from Zhu's genealogy.

Preserved by Feng Hanlong from Yiwu, Zhejiang Province

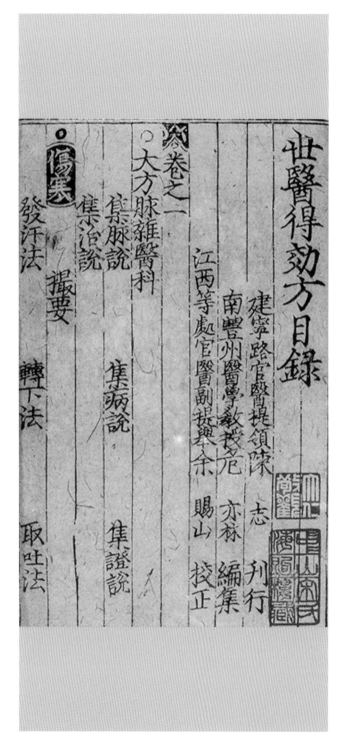

《世医得效方》书影

元

元至正五年陈志刊本。危亦林撰。书成于1337年。20卷。作者整理家传五世累积验方，并收集历代各科效方，按医学十三科编著成书。其第18卷专门论述正骨兼金镞科（即伤科），总结了14世纪我国骨伤科学的重要成就。

中国中医科学院图书馆藏

Book Photograph of *Shi Yi De Xiao Fang* (Family Prescriptions of Traditional Chinese Medicine)

Yuan Dynasty

This is the edition published by Chen Zhi. The author was Wei Yilin, who finished the book in 1337. There are 20 chapters. The author collected five generations' prescriptions of his family, as well as the effective prescriptions of the past dynasties. He compiled them into a book with 13 medical sectors. The 18th chapter mainly discussed department of traumatology, which summarized the significant achievements of orthopedics of Chinese Medicine in the 14th Century.

Preserved in Library of China Academy of Chinese Medical Sciences

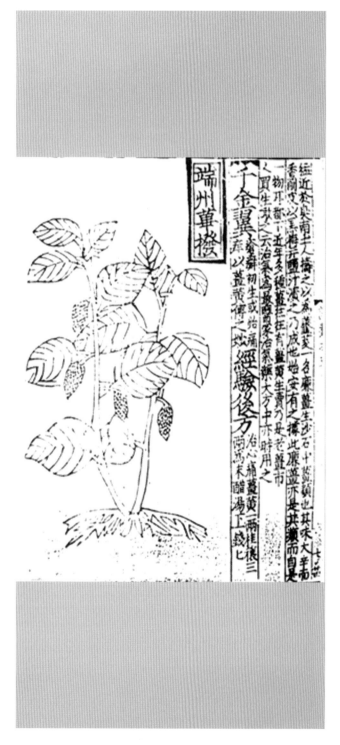

《证类本草》书影

宋

图为本书首刻本《大观本草》系统的南宋嘉定四年（1211）刘甲刻本。本书全称为《经史证类备急本草》，唐慎微撰。32卷。系据宋初《嘉祐补注本草》和《本草图经》两书汇集增益而成。收载药物1558种，多附药图，并记述药物的采集、炮制法等，兼录方剂3000多首。宋大观、政和、绍兴等年间数次校刊，其后历代传刻极多。本书历来为医家所重视，是研究宋以前本草学的重要文献。

首都图书馆藏

Book Photograph of *Zheng Lei Ben Cao* (Classified Materia Medica)

Song Dynasty

The picture is the block-printed edition by Liu Jia in the year 1211, which is one of the series of book named *Da Guan Ben Cao*, also the first block-printed version of *Zheng Lei Ben Cao*. The full name of this book is *Jing Shi Zheng Lei Bei Ji Ben Cao* written by Tang Shenwei, There are 32 chapters. This book grew out of *Jia You Bu Zhu Ben Cao* and *Ben Cao Tu Jing*, another two books of agrostology in early Song Dynasty. It collected 1,558 kinds of Chinese herbal medicines, most with pictures. It also described their gathering and manufacturing methods, as well as more than 3,000 prescriptions. This book was published many times during the Song Dynasty and the following dynasties. It was always regarded as the important medical document for researching agrostology before the Song Dynasty.

Preserved in Capital Library of China

《流注指要赋》书影

元

元《济生拔萃》本。金元医家窦默撰。内容以歌赋体扼要论述针灸诊治取穴之道。

中国中医科学院图书馆藏

Book Photograph of *Liu Zhu Zhi Yao Fu*

Yuan Dynasty

This book is from the medical series *Ji Sheng Ba Cui*. The author was Chinese physician Dou Mo in the Yuan Dynasty. It simply discusses treatment with acupuncture and moxibustion by the style of poetry.

Preserved in Library of China Academy of Chinese Medical Sciences

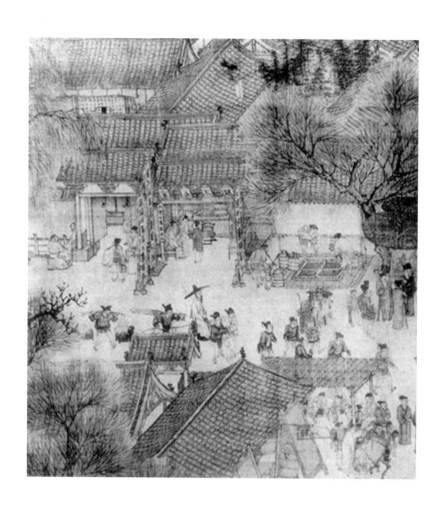

《清明上河图》中之"赵太丞家"

宋

《清明上河图》全图纵 24.8 厘米，横 528 厘米，为宋代张择端所绘的一幅名画，真实生动地反映了当时社会生活的场景。"赵太丞家"是其中的一部分，系开业医生的诊所兼药店。门前所立高大市招上书有"治酒所伤真方集香丸""大理中丸医肠胃冷"字样。

台北故宫博物院藏

Qing Ming Shang He Tu (Partial)

Song Dynasty

The vertical length of the painting *Qing Ming Shang He Tu* (Riverside Scene at Qingming Festival) is 24.8 cm, and its whole horizontal length is 528 cm. It is a famous painting by Zhang Zeduan in the Song Dynasty. It vividly reflects the scene of social life at that time. This preserved part called "Zhao Taicheng's House" depicts a clinic which was also a pharmacy. In front of the door, there are plaques with characters showing the medicines it sold.

Preserved in National Palace Museum

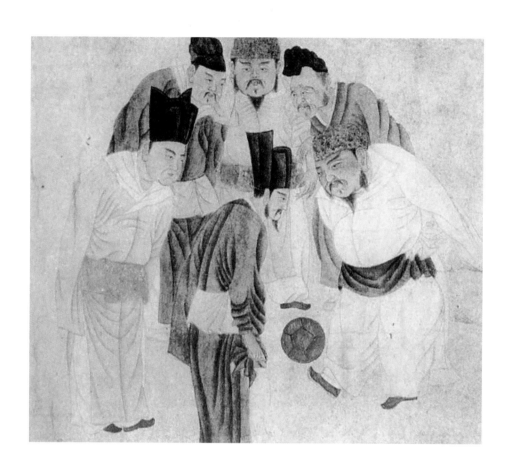

钱选《宋太宗蹴鞠图》

元

纵 28.6 厘米，横 56.3 厘米

设色。这幅画描绘了宋太祖赵匡胤（960—976 年在位）、宋太宗赵匡义（977—997 年在位）和近臣
赵普等一起蹴鞠玩乐的情景。

上海博物馆藏

Song Tai Zong Cu Ju Tu by Qian Xuan

Yuan Dynasty

Vertical Length 28.6 cm / Horizontal Length 56.3 cm

This painting depicts the scene of a Cuju game played by Zhao Kuangyin (the first emperor in the Song Dynasty from 960 to 976), Zhao Kuangyi (the second emperor in the Song Dynasty from 977 to 997), Zhao Pu (a courtier) and other people.

Preserved in Shanghai Museum

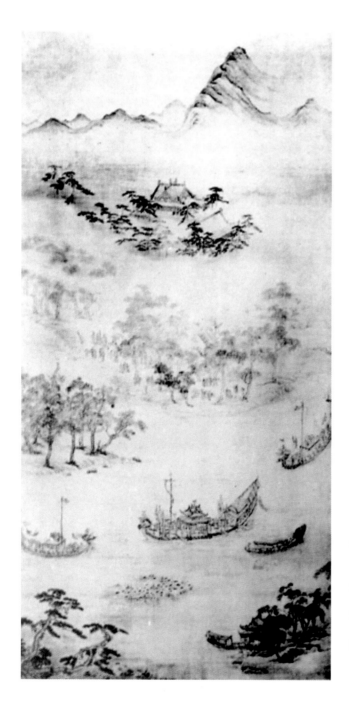

吴延晖《龙舟夺标图》

元

画家在尺幅之中，以精密、娴熟的艺术技巧，描绘了元人庞大的竞渡活动场景。

故宫博物院藏

Long Zhou Duo Biao Tu by Wu Yanhui

Yuan Dynasty

This painting shows us with skilled artistry a spectacular scene of dragon boat race in the Yuan Dynasty.

Preserved in The Palace Museum

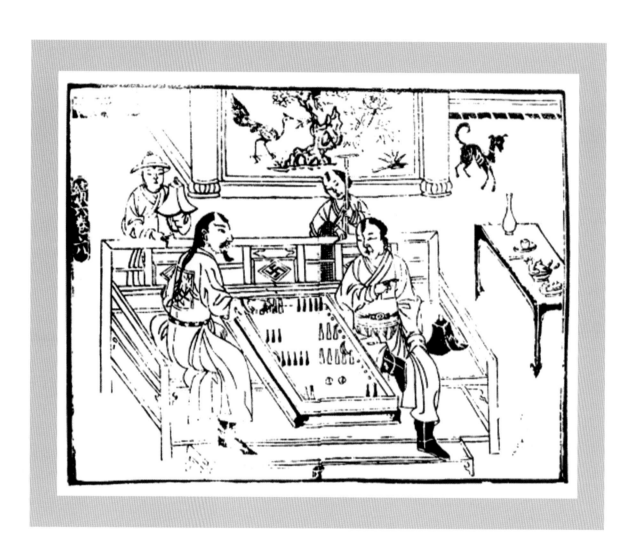

《事林广记·双陆图》

元

元至顺间建安椿庄书院刻本。《事林广记》42卷，12册，宋人陈元靓撰。图中描绘了两个蒙古装束的官员对局的情景。双陆局上有用牙形门和圆形花眼，并布有黑、白各十五枚双陆子和二骰子。榻后有两个蒙古装束的随从侍立。

中国国家图书馆藏

Shi Lin Guang Ji- Shuang Lu Tu

Yuan Dynasty

Compiled by Chen Yuanjing in the Song Dynasty, this book was the block-printed edition by Jian'an Chunzhuang Academy during the Yuan Dynasty (1330–1332). This painting is from *Shi Lin Guang Ji* (an encyclopedia-like book), which has 42 chapters and 12 volumes. This painting shows two Mongolian-dressed officials playing a game called Shuanglu. On the game table, there are crescent-like doors and round holes, as well as 15 black and 15 white pieces and two dices. Behind the seats, there are two servants standing there.

Preserved in National Library of China

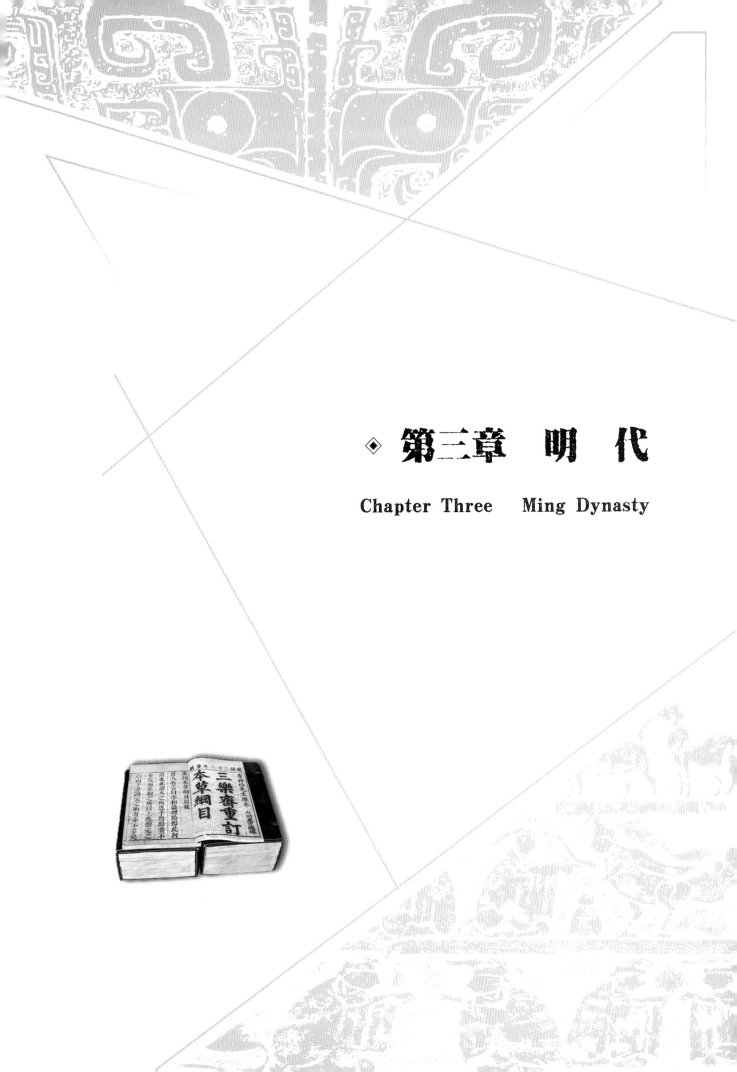

◈ 第三章　明　代

Chapter Three　　Ming Dynasty

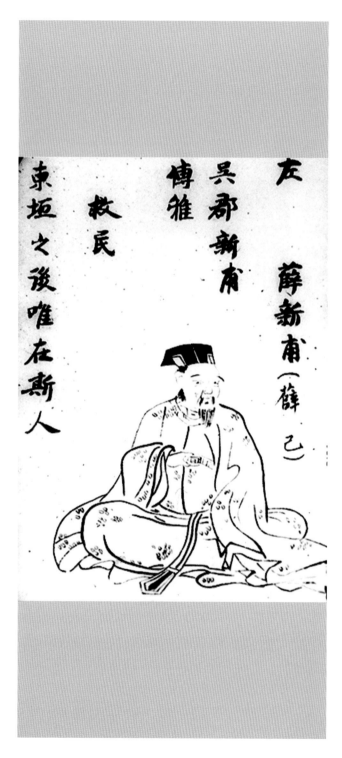

薛己木刻画像

明

薛己（1487—1559），明代医家。字新甫，号立斋。正德时选御医，擢南京院判，嘉靖间进院使，视篆南北两太医院，后致政归吴，徜徉丘垄，上下古今，研精覃思20年。（图为《医仙图赞》中薛己画像）

中国中医科学院图书馆藏

Wood Carving Portrait of Xue Ji

Ming Dynasty

Xue Ji (1487–1559) was a Chinese physician in the Ming Dynasty. His courtesy name was Xinfu, and his pseudonym was Lizhai. He was chosen as the Imperial Physician during the years of the reign of Emperor Zhengde and was Yuanpan (an official name) of Nanjing. During the years of the reign of Emperor Jiajing, he was Yuanshi, the chief of two major Imperial Hospitals at that time. Then he retired and returned to his native county, where he wandered in the fields, studied the past and present, and devoted himself to in-depth study in the following 20 years. This portrait of Xue Ji is from the book of *Yi Xian Tu Zan* (Pictures of Famous Doctors).

Preserved in Library of China Academy of Chinese Medical Sciences

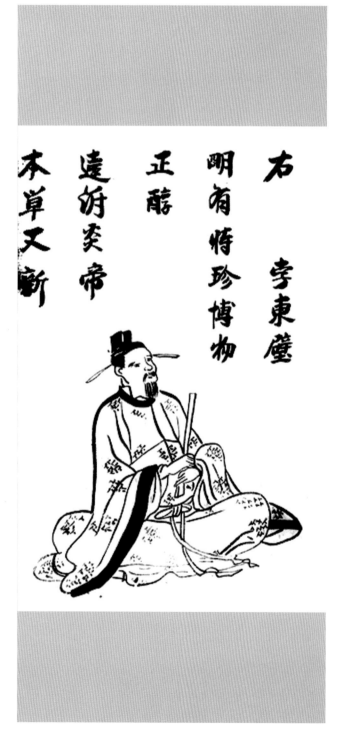

右　李東璧

明有持珍博物

正醇

遠游炎帝

本草又斬

李时珍术刻画像

明

李时珍（1518—1593），明代杰出医药学家。字东璧，晚号濒湖山人，蕲州（今湖北蕲春）人。曾掌楚王府良医所事，后曾供职于京师太医院。所著《本草纲目》一书，为古代医药学及博物学巨著。另著有《濒湖脉学》《奇经八脉考》及文学著作《所馆诗话》等书。（图为《医仙图赞》一书中之李时珍画像）

中国中医科学院图书馆藏

Wood Carving Portrait of Li Shizhen

Ming Dynasty

Li Shizhen(1518–1593) was an outstanding pharmacologist in the Ming Dynasty. His courtesy name was Dongbi, and his pseudonym in his old age was Binhu Shanren. He came from Qizhou (now Qichun County in Hubei Province). He was onced in charge of doctors of King Chu's Palace and then held a position in the Imperial Hospital of Beijing. He was the author of *Ben Cao Gang Mu*, which was a great work of both medical science and natural history in ancient China. He also wrote other medical books such as *Bin Hu Mai Xue*, *Qi Jing Ba Mai Kao*, and *Suo Guan Shi Hua*. This portrait of Li Shenzhen is from the book of *Yi Xian Tu Zan* (Pictures of Famous Doctors).

Preserved in Library of China Academy of Chinese Medical Sciences

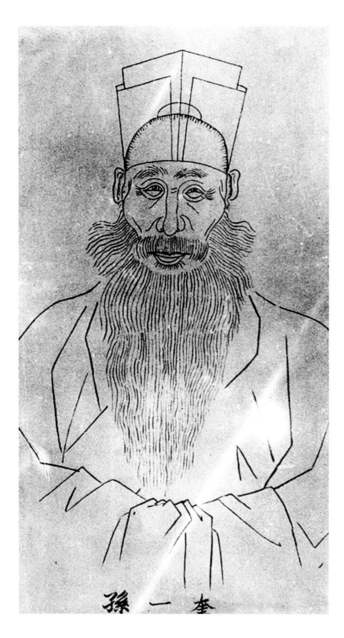

孙一奎木刻画像

明

孙一奎，明代医家。字文垣，号文宿，又号生生子，安徽休宁人。生活于嘉靖至万历年间（1522—1619），撰有《赤水玄珠》《孙文垣医案》等书。图为《赤水玄珠》一书中之孙氏木刻画像。

安徽中医药大学图书馆藏

Wood Carving Portrait of Sun Yikui

Ming Dynasty

Sun Yikui (1522–1619) was a physician in the Ming Dynasty. His courtesy name was Wenyuan, and his pseudonym was Wensu or Shengshengzi. He came from Xiuning County, Anhui Province. He wrote many medical books such as *Chi Shui Xuan Zhu* and *Sun Wen Yuan Yi An*. This wood carving portrait of him is from the book of *Chi Shui Xuan Zhu*.

Preserved in Library of Anhui University of Chinese Medicine

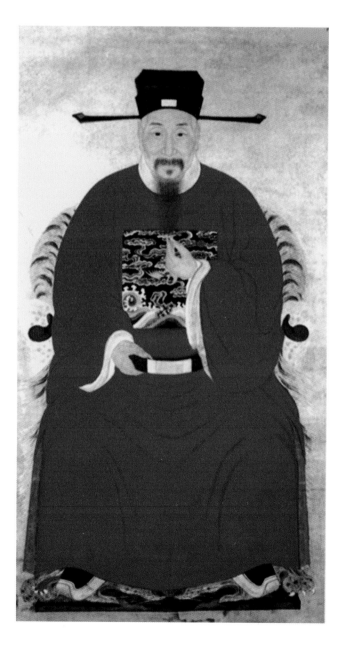

王肯堂画像

明

宽 75 厘米，高 130 厘米

王肯堂（1549—1613），明代医学家。字宇泰，号损庵，金坛（今属江苏）人。撰有《证治准绳》44 卷，并辑刻《古今医统正脉全书》，收明以前医书 44 种。金坛王氏家传。

中国医史博物馆藏

Portrait of Wang Kentang

Ming Dynasty

Width 75 cm/ Height 130 cm

Wang Kentang (1549–1613) was a medical scientist in the Ming Dynasty. His courtesy name was Yutai, and his pseudonym was Sun'an. He came from Jintan (now in Jiangsu Province). He was the author of *Zheng Zhi Zhun Sheng*, which has 44 chapters. He also compiled *Gu Jin Yi Tong Zheng Mai Quan Shu*, which collected 44 kinds of medical books before the Ming Dynasty. This portrait was an heirloom of Family Wang.

Preserved in Chinese Medical History Museum

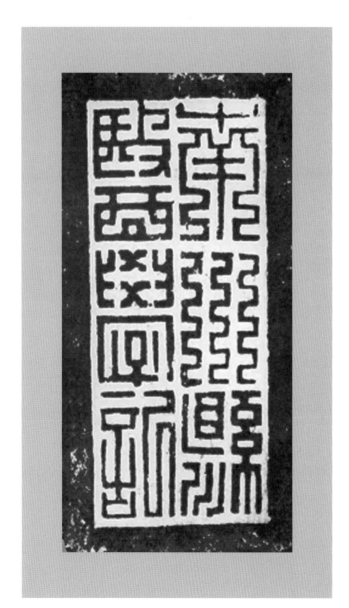

"南川县医学记"印蜕

明

原印：长 7.9 厘米，宽 4 厘米，印面厚 1.1 厘米

洪武三十五年十二月礼部造，为地方政府印记。

四川大学博物馆藏

Stamp of Official Seal

Ming Dynasty

The Original Seal: Length 7.9 cm/ Width 4 cm/
Surface Thickness 1.1 cm

The characters on the seal are "Nan Chuan
Xian Yi Xue Ji". It was made by the Ministry
of Rites in December of the 35th year of the
reign of Emperor Zhu Yuanzhang for the local
government of Nanchuan County, Sichuan
Province.

Preserved in Sichuan University Museum

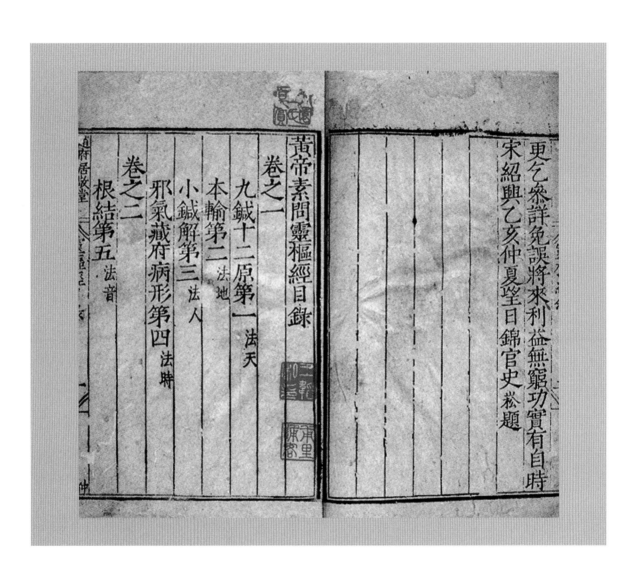

《黄帝内经·灵枢》书影

明

嘉靖间赵府居敬堂刊本。本书一名《针经》，古时亦称《九卷》《九灵》，与《素问》合称《黄帝内经》。
本书性质与《素问》相似，但其内容偏于针灸论述较多。原书在晋唐时流传不广，至宋代史崧以家藏旧
本校刊，分成 24 卷，共 81 篇，遂广泛流传。

中国中医科学院图书馆藏

Book Photograph of *Huang Di Nei Jing- Ling Shu*

Ming Dynasty

It was the edition by Zhaofu Ju Jing Tang (name of a publishing house) during the reign of Emperor Jiajing. This book was once called *Zhen Jing*, as well as *Jiu Juan* or *Jiu Ling* in ancient China. This book and another book *Su Wen* are collectively called the famous ancient Chinese medical book *Huang Di Nei Jing* (Inner Canon of the Yellow Emperor). *Ling Shu* and *Su Wen* are very similar in style, but this one mainly discusses acupuncture and moxibustion. The original book was not that popular in the Jin and Tang Dynasties. In the Song Dynasty, Shi Song got it published again according to his family collection and divided it into 24 chapters and 81 articles, which were widely spread from then on. Preserved in Library of China Academy of Chinese Medical Sciences

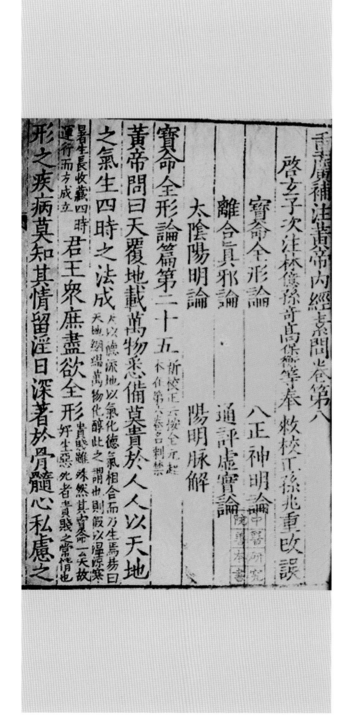

《黄帝内经·素问》书影

明

顾从德本。《素问》乃《黄帝内经》中之一部，
是现存最早的中医理论著作之一，约成书于
战国时期。非一人一时之作，黄帝乃托名。
本书为中医最重要的经典著作之一。

中国中医科学院图书馆藏

Book Photograph of *Huang Di Nei Jing- Su Wen*

Ming Dynasty

This copy is of Gu Congde's edition. *Su Wen* (Plain Questions) is one part of *Huang Di Nei Jing*. It is one of the earliest works about traditional Chinese medical theories. This book was completed in about the Warring States Period. Actually it was not written by just one author in one period. It is one of the most important books of traditional Chinese medicine.

Preserved the Library of China Academy of Chinese Medical Sciences

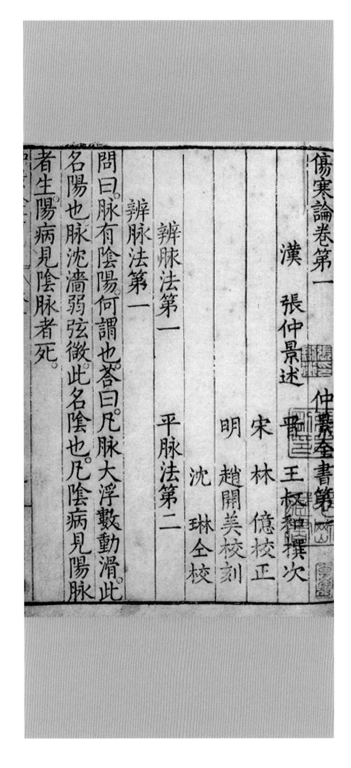

《伤寒论》书影

明

万历二十七年（1599）海虞赵开美刻本。本书系张仲景所著《伤寒杂病论》一书中论治伤寒的部分。今传本为晋代王叔和编次，宋代林亿校正，全书 10 卷，22 篇。书中以六经为辨证论治纲领，归纳总结了外感热病的发生、发展、转归的全过程，并系统论述了其诊断、辨证与治疗。本书与《金匮要略》所确立的辨证论治原则，对后世有深远的影响。

中国中医科学院图书馆藏

Book Photograph of *Shang Han Lun*

Ming Dynasty

This copy of *Shang Han Lun* (Treatise on Febrile Diseases) is of the block-printed edition by Zhao Kaimei in 1599. Mainly discussing exogenous febrile diseases, this book was part of *Shang Han Za Bing Lun* written by Zhang Zhongjing. It was compiled by Wang Shuhe in the Jin Dynasty and calibrated by Lin Yi in the Song Dynasty. There are 10 chapters and 22 articles. Based on the theories of "Liu Jing" (six classics), this book summarizes the whole process of exogenous febrile diseases and systematically discusses the diagnosis analysis and treatment of the diseases. Together with *Jin Gui Yao Lüe* (Medical Treasures of Golden Chamber), the principles of treating diseases in this book have exerted a great influence on later generations.

Preserved in Library of China Academy of Chinese Medical Sciences

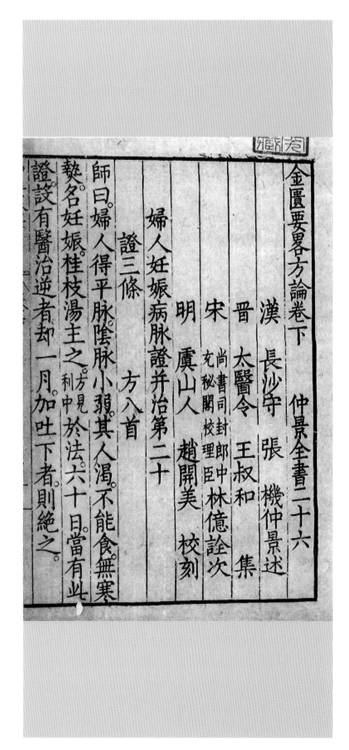

《金匮要略》书影

明

万历二十七年（1599）海虞赵开美刻本。《金
匮要略方论》简称《金匮要略》，系张仲景
所著《伤寒杂病论》中论治杂病部分。今传
本系晋代王叔和编次、宋代孙奇等根据王洙
发现的残本校定而成。全书共25篇，总结了
我国东汉以前的丰富诊疗经验，是奠定我国
临证医学基础的重要古典医籍之一。

中国中医科学院图书馆藏

Book Photograph of *Jin Gui Yao Lüe*

Ming Dynasty

This copy of *Jin Gui Yao Lüe* (Medical Treasures of Golden Chamber) is of the block-printed edition by Zhao Kaimei in 1599. Its full name is *Jin Gui Yao Lüe Fang Lun*. Mainly discussing the miscellaneous diseases, this book was part of *Shang Han Za Bing Lun* written by Zhang Zhongjing. It was compiled by Wang Shuhe in the Jin Dynasty, and proofread by Sun Qi in the Song Dynasty according to an incomplete copy found by Wang Zhu. This book contains 25 articles summarizing the rich treatment experience before the Eastern Han Dynasty. It is one of the important medical classics, which laid the foundation for Chinese clinical medicine.

Preserved in Library of China Academy of Chinese Medical Sciences

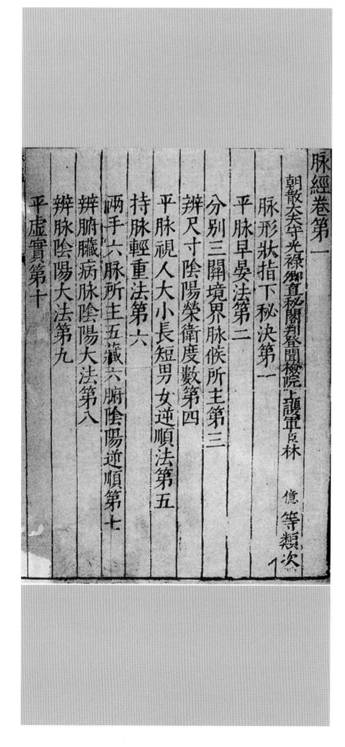

《脉经》书影

明

《医统正脉》本。由晋代王叔和总结前人的脉学内容而写成，共 10 卷，是我国现存最早的脉学专著。此书将脉象归纳为 24 种类型，保存了晋以前的脉学文献，是后世中医脉学发展的重要基础。

中国中医科学院图书馆藏

Book Photograph of *Mai Jing*

Ming Dynasty

Yi Tong Zheng Mai was the documentary edition of this book. *Mai Jing* (the Book of Pulse) was written by Wang Shuhe in the Jin Dynasty, who summarized the sphygmology of the predecessors in 10 chapters. And it is the earliest Chinese monograph in this field. The book has grouped the pulse manifestations into 24 types and accumulated the relevant literature before the Jin Dynasty. It is an important foundation for the later development of sphygmology in traditional Chinese medicine.

Preserved in Library of China Academy of Chinese Medical Sciences

唐王燾先生外臺秘要方第一卷

宋朝散大夫守光祿卿直秘閣判登聞簡院上護軍臣林億等
上進

中憲大夫徽州府知府 富湖玉井陸錫明校閱

新安後學程衍道敬逼父訂梓

諸論傷寒八家合一十六首

陰陽大論云春氣温和夏氣著熱秋氣清凉冬氣凛冽此
則四時正氣之序也冬時嚴寒萬額深藏君子周密則不
傷於寒觸冒之者乃名傷寒耳其傷於四時之氣皆能為
病以傷寒為毒者以其最成殺癘之氣也中而即病者名
日傷寒不即病者寒毒藏於肌膚中至春變為温病至夏

《外台秘要》书影

明

崇祯庚辰年（1640）新安程衍道刻本。本书
为王焘约撰于752年，40卷，包括临证各
科与药物等共1104门，均先论后方，载方
6000余首，各详注出处。此书汇集了初唐
以前数十种医学著作，在保存古代医学文献
方面做出了较大贡献。

中国中医科学院图书馆藏

Book Photograph of *Wai Tai Mi Yao*

Ming Dynasty

This book was the block-printed edition made by Cheng Yandao in 1640. The book was written by Wang Tao in about 752. There are 40 chapters and 1,104 subjects, including clinical diseases and medicines. There are more than 6,000 prescriptions, each of which had clear references. This book collected dozens of medical works before the early Tang Dynasty, and has made a great contribution to the preservation of ancient medical literature.

Preserved in Library of China Academy of Chinese Medical Sciences

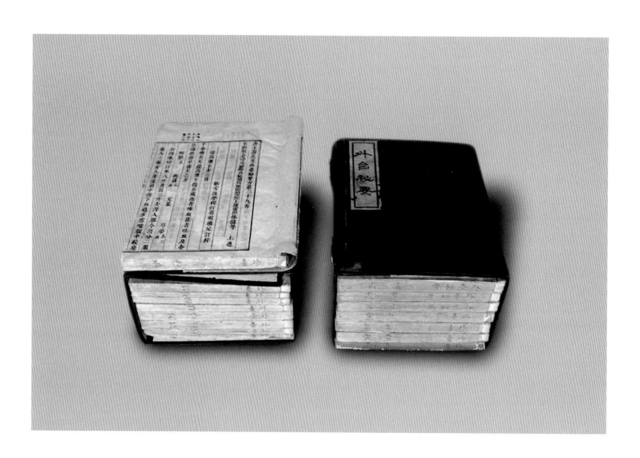

《外台秘要》四十卷

明

明代崇祯十三年（1640），新安程衍道经余居刻本。唐代王焘撰，明代程衍道（敬通）校，日本山胁尚德补校。3 函 22 册。保存完整。陕西中医药大学图书馆调拨。

陕西医史博物馆藏

Wai Tai Mi Yao (40 Chapters)

Ming Dynasty

It is the block-printed edition of Cheng Yandao in 1640. The book was written by Wang Tao in the Tang Dynasty, proofread by Cheng Yandao in the Ming Dynasty, and re-proofread by Yamawaki from Japan. There are 3 sets and 22 volumes. The books are in complete condition and are allocated from the Library of Shaanxi University of Chinese Medicine.

Preserved in Shaanxi Museum of Medical History

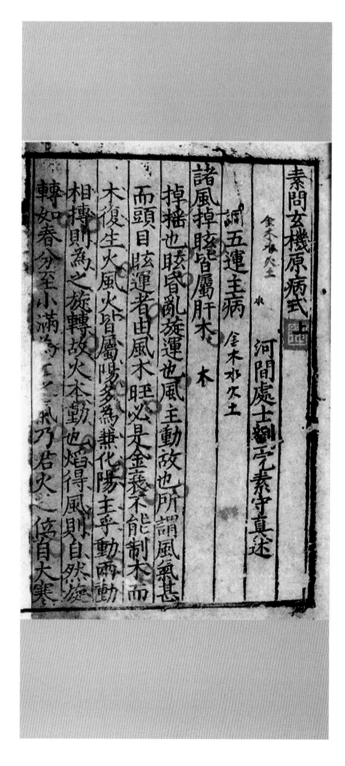

《素问玄机原病式》书影

明

《医统正脉》本。金代刘完素撰，约成书于
1152年。1卷。书中将《素问·至真要大论》
中的"病机十九条"依据五运六气主病整理
归纳为十一条病机，共277字。

中国中医科学院图书馆藏

Book Photograph of *Su Wen Xuan Ji Yuan Bing Shi*

Ming Dynasty

Yi Tong Zheng Mai was the documentary edition of this book. The book was written by Liu Wansu in the Jin Dynasty and completed in about 1152. There is only 1 chapter in this book, which has summarized 11 types of pathogenesis in 277 characters based on the 19 types of pathogenesis in *Su Wen–Zhi Zhen Yao Da Lun*, according to five elements' motion and six kinds of natural factors of diseases.

Preserved in Library of China Academy of Chinese Medical Sciences

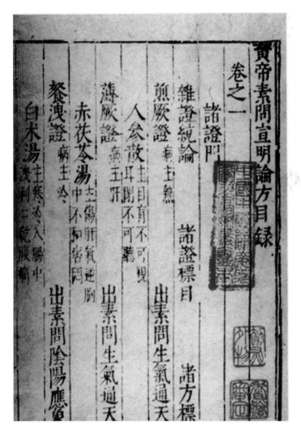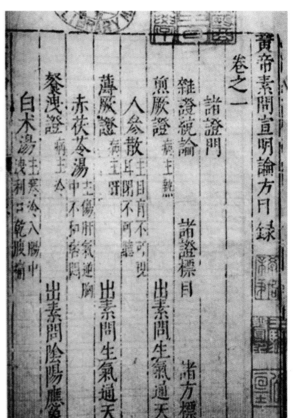

《黄帝素问宣明论方》书影

明

《医统正脉》本。金代刘完素撰于大定十二年（1172）。3卷（一作15卷）。对《素问》所述若干病症予以阐发，并补充方治。

中国中医科学院图书馆藏

Book Photograph of *Huang Di Su Wen Xuan Ming Lun Fang*

Ming Dynasty

Yi Tong Zheng Mai was the documentary edition of this book. It was written by Liu Wansu in the Jin Dynasty (1172). The book has 3 chapters (or 15 chapters in an other edition). It expounds some diseases described in *Su Wen* (Plain Questions), and supplements some treatment prescriptions.

Preserved in Library of China Academy of Chinese Medical Sciences

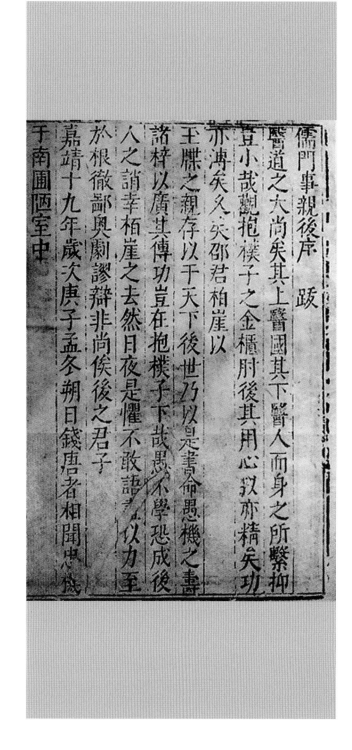

《儒门事亲》书影

明

《医统正脉》本。金代张子和与麻知几、常仲明等辑著，约成书于13世纪20年代。15卷。内容为阐述运用汗、吐、下三法治病的理论和临诊经验，并列举了各类病症200多例来说明其攻邪治法的疗效。

中国中医科学院图书馆藏

Book Photograph of *Ru Men Shi Qin*

Ming Dynasty

Yi Tong Zheng Mai was the documentary edition of this book. The book *Ru Men Shi Qin* (Confucian's Duties to Their Parents) was written by Zhang Zihe, Ma Zhiji, Chang Zhongming and so on in the Jin Dynasty. It was completed in the 1220s. There are 15 chapters in this book, which elaborates the theory and clinical experience of treating illnesses by the means of sweat, vomitting and diarrhea. It also enumerates more than 200 cases to illustrate the curative effect.

Preserved in Library of China Academy of Chinese Medical Sciences

脾胃論卷上

脾胃虛實傳變論

新安 吳中珩 校

五藏別論云胃大腸小腸三焦膀胱此五者天氣之
所生也其氣象天故瀉而不藏此受五藏濁氣名曰
傳化之府此不能久留輸瀉者也所謂五藏者藏精
氣而不瀉也故滿而不能實六腑者傳化物而不藏
故實而不能滿所以然者水穀入口則胃實而腸虛
食下則腸實而胃虛故曰實而不滿滿而不實也陰
陽應象大論云穀氣通於脾六經爲川腸胃爲海九

《脾胃论》书影

明

《医统正脉》本。金元医家李杲著于1249年。
3卷。《脾胃论》主要论述了脾胃虚弱所致
诸病及处方用药法。

中国中医科学院图书馆藏

Book Photograph of *Pi Wei Lun*

Ming Dynasty

Yi Tong Zheng Mai was the documentary edition of this book. The book *Pi Wei Lun* (Treatise on the Spleen and Stomach) was written in 1249 by Li Gao, a physician in the Jin and Yuan Dynasties. There are 3 chapters. It mainly discusses various diseases caused by the weakness of spleen and stomach, as well as the prescriptions and instructions.

Preserved in Library of China Academy of Chinese Medical Sciences

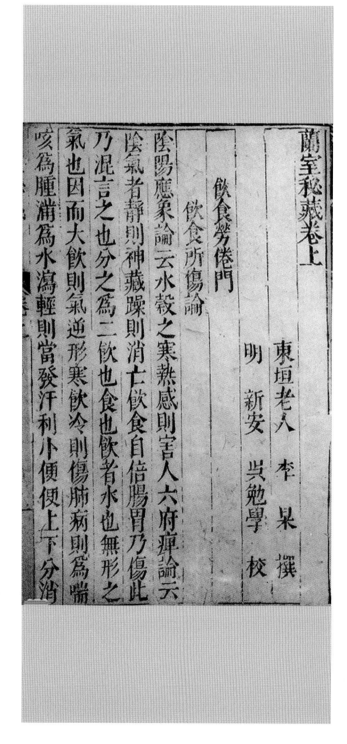

兰室秘藏卷上

東垣老人 李杲 撰

明 新安 吳勉學 校

飲食勞倦門

飲食所傷論

陰陽應象論云水穀之寒熱感則害人六府痺論云

陰陽者靜則神藏躁則消亡飲食自倍腸胃乃傷此

乃混言之也分之爲二飲也食也飲者水也無形之

氣也因而大飲則氣逆形寒飲冷則傷肺病則爲喘

咳爲腫滿爲水瀉輕則當發汗利小便便上下分消

《兰室秘藏》书影

明

《医统正脉》本。李杲著。首刊于元至元

十三年（1276）。3卷。分20门。全书以

内科杂病为主，兼及临证各科。内科杂病中

又以脾胃病症为重点，载方280首。

中国中医科学院图书馆藏

Book Photograph of *Lan Shi Mi Zang*

Ming Dynasty

Yi Tong Zheng Mai was the documentary edition of this book. *Lan Shi Mi Zang* (Secret Book of Orchid Chamber) was written by Li Gao. The first edition was published in 1276. There are 3 chapters and 20 subjects. This book mainly introduces the internal miscellaneous diseases and clinical subjects, with the focus on diseases of spleen and stomach, and also records 280 prescriptions.

Preserved in Library of China Academy of Chinese Medical Sciences

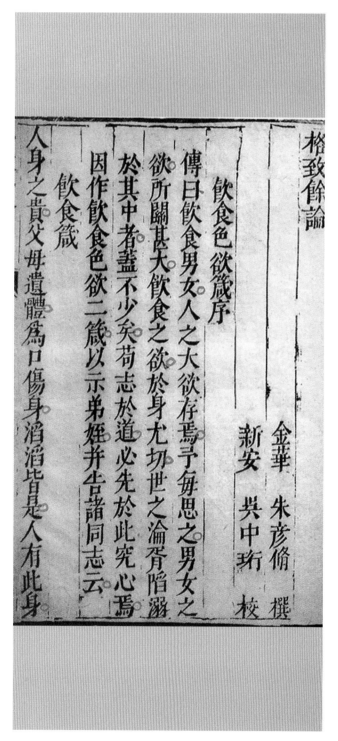

人身之貴父母遺體爲口傷身滔滔皆是人有此身

飲食箴

因作飲食色欲二箴以示弟姪并告諸同志云

於其中者蓋不少矣苟志於道必先於此究心焉

欲所關其大飲食之欲於身尤切世之淪胥陷溺

傅曰飲食男女人之大欲存焉予每思之男女之

飲食色欲箴序

格致餘論　　金華　朱彥修　撰

　　　　　　新安　吳中珩　校

《格致余论》书影

明

《医统正脉》本。朱震亨撰于至正七年

（1347）。全书载 40 余篇医论，较充分地

反映了朱氏倡导的补阴派的学术思想。

中国中医科学院图书馆藏

Book Photograph of *Ge Zhi Yu Lun*

Ming Dynasty

Yi Tong Zheng Mai was the documentary edition of this book. *Ge Zhi Yu Lun* (Further Discourses on the Properties of Things) was written by Zhu Zhenheng in 1347. The book contains more than 40 medical articles and fully reflects Zhu's academic ideas of tonifying Yin.

Preserved in Library of China Academy of Chinese Medical Sciences

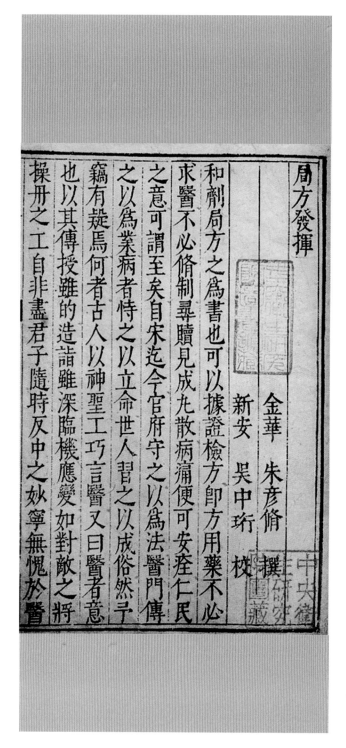

《局方发挥》书影

明

《医统正脉》本。朱震亨约撰于 14 世纪中期。

1 卷。作者鉴于《和剂局方》一书中存在的

偏颇，列举其 31 条并逐一评论。

中国中医科学院图书馆藏

Book Photograph of *Ju Fang Fa Hui*

Ming Dynasty

Yi Tong Zheng Mai was the documentary edition of this book. *Ju Fang Fa Hui* (Elaboration of Dispensary Formulas) was written by Zhu Zhenheng in the mid-14th Century. The book contains only 1 volume. In view of some problems in the book *He Ji Ju Fang*, the author cited 31 prescriptions and commented on them one by one.

Preserved in Library of China Academy of Chinese Medical Sciences

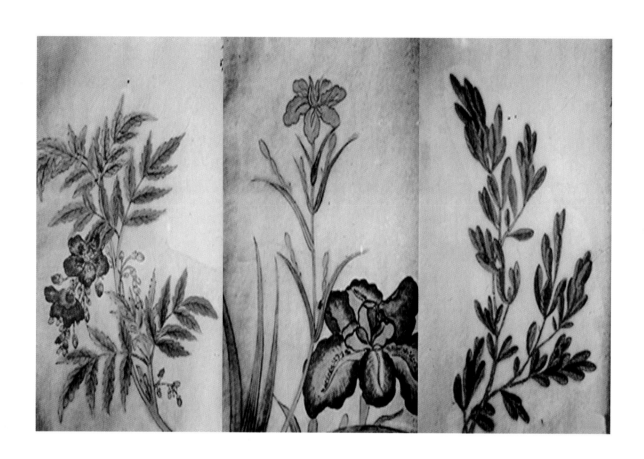

《履巉岩本草》书影

明

摹宋绘本。本书为我国本草史上流传不多的彩绘图谱之一。南宋画家、医药爱好者王介编绘于1220年。

3卷。原绘药图206幅，今实有202幅。原书已佚，今存明摹绘本。图为该书的凌霄花、山姜花与扁竹

三图。

首都图书馆藏

Book Photograph of *Lü Chan Yan Ben Cao*

Ming Dynasty

The book is the facsimile copy of the painting in the Song Dynasty. The book *Lü Chan Yan Ben Cao* (Herbage on Precipitous Rock) is one of the few colored picture collections in the history of agrostology. It was compiled and painted by Wang Jie in 1220, who was an artist and medical amateur in the Southern Song Dynasty. There are 3 chapters. There were 206 original herbal paintings, but now only 202 remain. The original book is missing. The three pictures are trumpet creeper, Japanese galangal flower and flat bamboo from this book.

Preserved in Capital Library of China

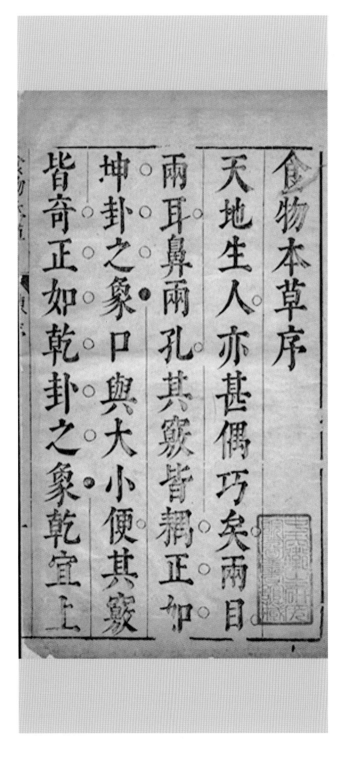

《食物本草》书影

明

成书于1621年，明代崇祯十五年壬午（1642）刻本。22卷。元代李杲编辑，明代李时珍参订。本草著作。共载食物1682条。前4卷为水部，载水750余味，包括37处名水，650处名泉，为介绍泉水功用集成之作。其余各卷之资料，多取自《本草纲目》，然鳞部、介部等处亦有新增之品。全书内容丰富，为古代食物本草之冠。

中国中医科学院图书馆藏

Book Photograph of *Shi Wu Ben Cao*

Ming Dynasty

Shi Wu Ben Cao (Food and Herbal Medicine) was completed in 1621 and published in the block-printed edition in 1642. There are 22 chapters. It was compiled by Li Gao in the Yuan Dynasty and revised by Li Shizhen in the Ming Dynasty. This book is a famous work in Chinese herbalism, with 1,682 items of food. The first 4 volumes are about water, and contained more than 750 flavors of water, including 37 famous sites of water and 650 famous springs. It is an integrated work introducing the functions of springs. The rest volumes were mostly derived from the *Ben Cao Gang Mu*, but there are also some supplements in sectors Lin and Jie. Rich in content, this book is the best in respect of the ancient Chinese food and herbal medicine.

Preserved in Library of China Academy of Chinese Medical Sciences

太平聖惠方卷第六十七　方九十五門　共計一百字九道

治從高臨下傷折諸方　八

治從高臨破骨傷筋諸方　一遍

治跌折破骨傷筋諸方　二

治一切傷折惡血不散諸方

治墜落車馬傷折諸方　八道

治馬墜諸方　二十四道

治壓笮墜墮內損諸方　七道

治打撲損諸方　二十二道

治傷折疼痛諸方　二十二道

治墜損吐唾血出諸方　置

治一切傷折煩悶諸方　四道

治一切傷折淋熨諸方　二十二道

治被打損肢中有瘀血諸方　二十四道

治從高墜下落馬墜車輾著跌撲骨碎筋傷內損惡血攻心悶絶坐臥不安宜先須椒摩排正筋骨後宜服止痛散血蒲黃散

治一切傷折膏茶諸方　二十三道

治一切傷折止痛生肌諸方　八道

治一切傷折疼痛貼熁諸方　二道

蒲黃二兩　　當歸三兩　　桂心三分　　延胡索一兩

《太平圣惠方》书影

明

日本1514年抄本。北宋王怀隐等人根据宋太宗亲藏验方千余首及当时医局所藏各家验方编纂而成。始编于太平兴国三年（978）。全书共分1670门，方16834首，并保存了不少已佚医书的内容。

中国中医科学院图书馆藏

Book Photograph of *Tai Ping Sheng Hui Fang*

Ming Dynasty

Tai Ping Sheng Hui Fang (Peaceful Holy Benevolent Prescriptions) is the Japanese hand copy version in 1514. The original book was first compiled in 978 by Wang Huaiyin of the Northern Song Dynasty according to more than a thousand prescriptions collected by Emperor Taizong of Song and those by the medical institutions at that time. The book has 1,670 categories and 16,834 prescriptions, including the contents of many lost medical books.

Preserved in Library of China Academy of Chinese Medical Sciences

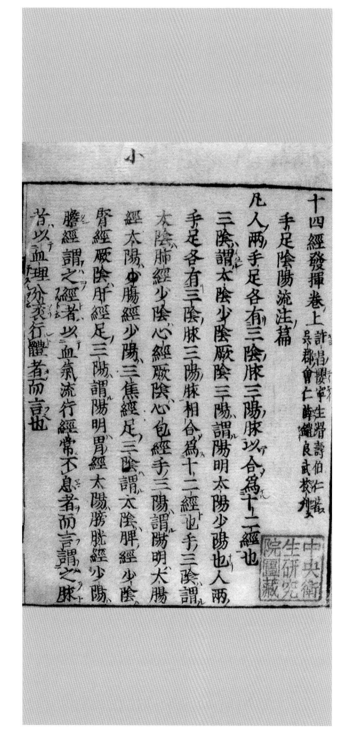

《十四经发挥》书影

明

明刊本。元代滑寿编著。书成于至正元年
（1341）。3卷。其为论述经络学说的专著。

中国中医科学院图书馆藏

Book Photograph of *Shi Si Jing Fa Hui*

Ming Dynasty

The book is the block-printed edition in the Ming Dynasty. *Shi Si Jing Fa Hui* (Elaboration of the Fourteen Channels) was compiled by Hua Shou of the Yuan Dynasty in 1341. Consisting of 3 chapters, it is a monograph about meridian theory. Preserved in Library of China Academy of Chinese Medical Sciences

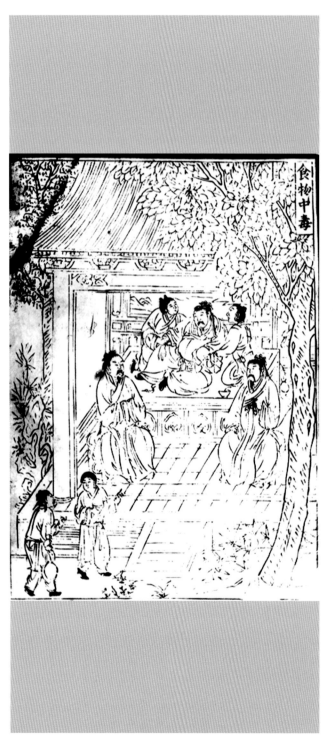

《饮膳正要》书影

明

明经厂刊本。元代饮膳太医、蒙古族营养学家忽思慧与大臣普兰奚编撰。3卷。刊于天历三年（1330）。本书系作者任职期间对食物营养、饮食卫生及其他有关知识的总结，是现存最早的营养学专著。书中附图168幅。

中国中医科学院图书馆藏

Book Photograph of *Yin Shan Zheng Yao*

Ming Dynasty

It is the factory block-printed edition in the Ming Dynasty. This three-chapter book named *Yin Shan Zheng Yao* (Principles of Correct Diet) was compiled by Hu Sihui, an imperial diet doctor and Mongolian nutritionist, and Pu Lanxi, a Minister in the Yuan Dynasty. It was published in 1330. It summarizes the food nutrition, food hygiene and other related knowledge accumulated during the tenure of the authors, and is the earliest monograph on nutrition. The book also includes 168 pictures.

Preserved in Library of China Academy of Chinese Medical Sciences

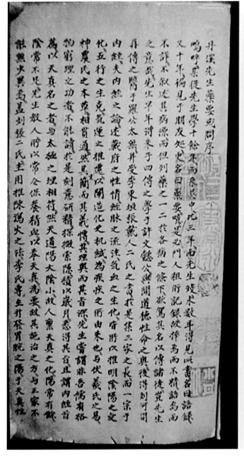

《丹溪先生药要或问》书影

明

明抄本。明代医家赵良仁撰。2卷。赵氏，字以德，号云居，江浦人，丹溪弟子，精医术。他感于《丹溪药要》一书有简略草率之嫌，乃据此设为问答，借以阐发丹溪的学术思想，并间附自己之医案。该抄本今存风证至小儿赤溜共128条。左图为书中赵氏自序，右图为卷上之一页。本抄本为该书仅存之孤本。

史常永供稿

Book Photograph of *Dan Xi Xian Sheng Yao Yao Huo Wen*

Ming Dynasty

The book is the hand–copied edition in the Ming Dynasty. *Dan Xi Xian Sheng Yao Yao Huo Wen* (Questions and Answers of Danxi Medical Principles) is a two-chapter book compiled in the Ming Dynasty by doctor Zhao Liangren, who was a medical expert of Danxi, a school of thought in ancient China. Considering the curtness of *Dan Xi Yao Yao* (Danxi Medical Principles), Zhao set questions and answers to elucidate Danxi's thought and attached his own medical cases. This hand-copied book includes 128 diseases. The left picture is the self-introduction of Zhao, and the right picture is one of the pages from Chapter I. This transcript is the only existing copy of the book.

Provided by Shi Changyong

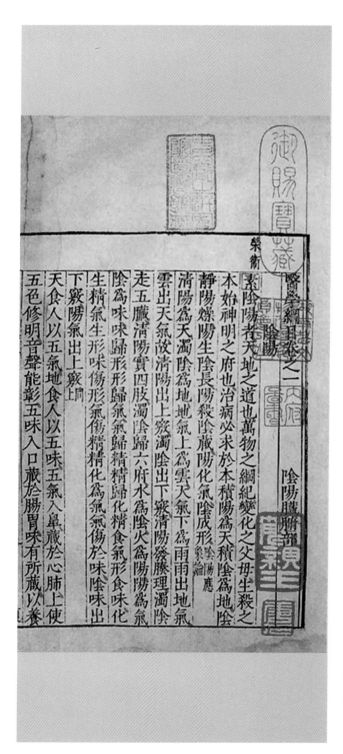

《医学纲目》书影

明

明刊本。明初医家楼英撰。40 卷。初刊于
嘉靖四十四年（1565）。本书将 600 多种
常见病症按部类分列叙述。

中国中医科学院图书馆藏

Book Photograph of *Yi Xue Gang Mu*

Ming Dynasty

The book is the block-printed edition in the Ming Dynasty.This 40-chapter book *Yi Xue Gang Mu* (Compendium of Medicine) was compiled by doctor Lou Ying in the early Ming Dynasty. It was first published in 1565. In this book, more than 600 common diseases are described by categories.

Preserved in Library of China Academy of Chinese Medical Sciences

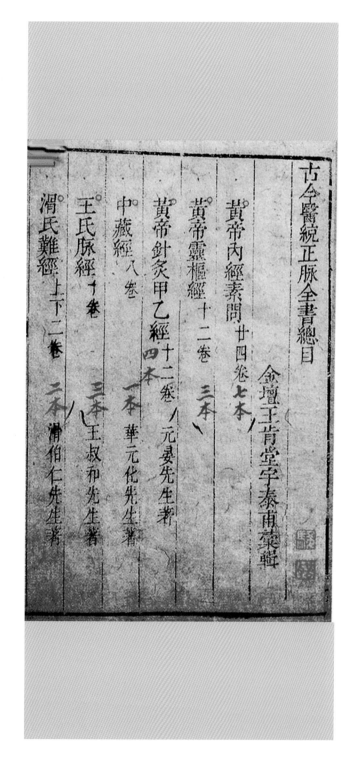

《古今医统正脉全书》书影

明

万历刊本。王肯堂汇辑，初刊于万历二十九年（1601），是现存较早的古代大型医学丛书，汇辑医书44种。

中国中医科学院图书馆藏

Book Photograph of *Gu Jin Yi Tong Zheng Mai Quan Shu*

Ming Dynasty

The book is block-printed edition in the reign of Emperor Wanli. The book *Gu Jin Yi Tong Zheng Mai Quan Shu* (Encyclopedia of Ancient and Modern Medical Systems) was compiled by Wang Kentang and first published in 1601. Including 44 medical books, it is the earliest existing multi-volume medical book series.

Preserved in Library of China Academy of Chinese Medical Sciences

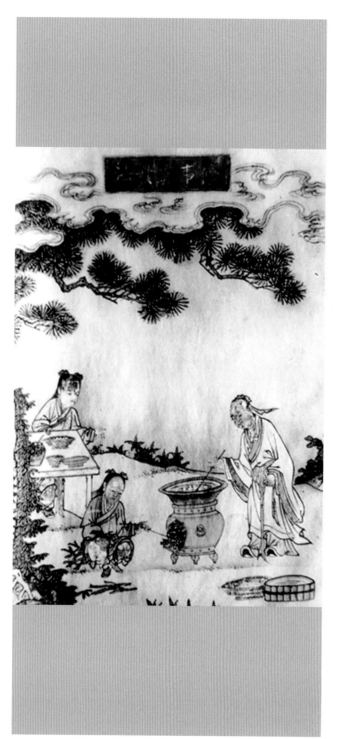

《本草品汇精要》书影

明

太医院院判刘文泰等奉命撰修。42 卷。
书成于弘治十八年（1505）。图为首都图
书馆藏明代弘治本副本。全书共收载药物
1815 种，原书有王世昌等 8 名画师所绘的
1358 幅五彩工笔药图，甚为精美。原书编
成后因故未得刊行而藏于内府。

首都图书馆藏

Book Photograph of *Ben Cao Pin Hui Jing Yao*

Ming Dynasty

The book *Ben Cao Pin Hui Jing Yao* (Concise Herbal Foundation Compilation) was compiled and revised by Liu Wentai under the instruction of the Imperial Hospital. It has 42 chapters and was finished in 1505. The picture is a copy of the Hongzhi edition of the book preserved in Capital Library of China. Totally 1,815 medicines are recorded in the book, which has 1,358 exquisite colored meticulous herb pictures painted by 8 famous artists like Wang Shichang and so on. When it was finished, for some reasons, it was not published but preserved in the imperial storehouse.

Preserved in Capital Library of China

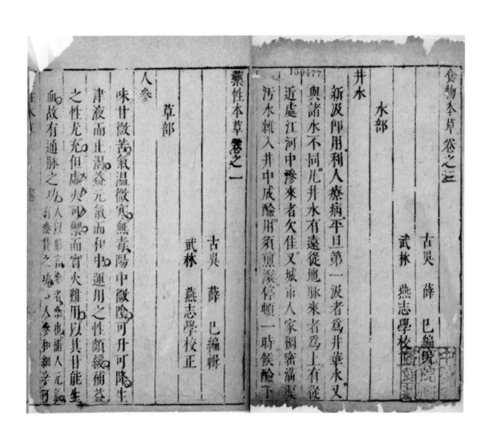

《本草约言》

明

明代木刻本。成书于 1520 年。4 卷。明代薛己编辑，燕志学校正。本草学专著。全书由《药性本草》《食物本草》两部分组成。此本《药性本草》首列"医学启源""药性旨要"，后分草、木、果、菜、米谷、金石、人、禽兽、虫草等 9 部，收药 287 种；《食物本草》则存水、谷、菜、果、禽、兽、鱼、味 8 部，存药 388 种，全书共存药约 675 种。论取简约，故名"约言"。

中国中医科学院图书馆藏

Ben Cao Yue Yan

Ming Dynasty

The book is the woodblock edition in the Ming Dynasty. *Ben Cao Yue Yan* (Herbal Brief Descriptions) is a four-chapter book finished in 1520, compiled by Xue Ji and revised by Yan Zhixue. It is a herbal monograph consisting two books *Yao Xing Ben Cao* (Medicinal Herbal) and *Shi Wu Ben Cao* (Food Herbal). "Medical Source" and "Medicinal Elements" were first listed in *Yao Xing Ben Cao*, which has recorded 287 kinds of medicines in nine categories namely grass, wood, fruit, vegetable, grain, stone, people, animal and Chinese caterpillar fungus. *Shi Wu Ben Cao* has 388 kinds of medicines in eight categories such as water, grain, vegetable, fruit, poultry, animal, fish and flavor. There are totally 675 medicines recorded in it. Because of concise introductions, the book was name as it is.

Preserved in Library of China Academy of Chinese Medical Sciences

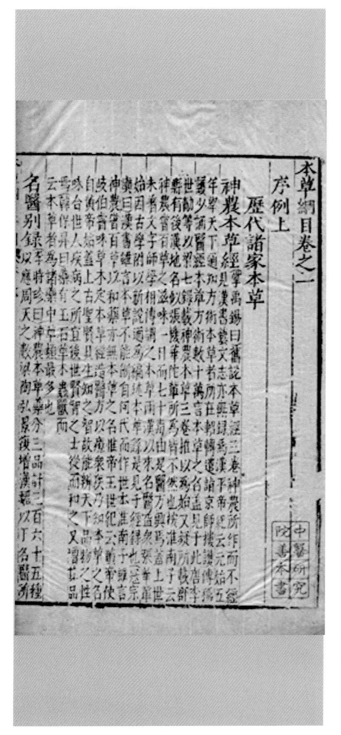

《本草纲目》

明

明万历十八年庚寅（1590）金陵刻本。成书于 1578 年。52 卷。明代李时珍编辑，李建中、李建元校正。本草学专著。卷 1、2 "序例" 述本草要籍与药性理论，"历代诸家本草" 介绍明以前主要本草 41 种。卷 3、4 为 "百病主治药"。卷 5~52 为各论，收药 1892 种，附图 1109 种。收药以《证类本草》为蓝本，新增药物 374 种。本书为明代本草集成之作，收药之众，内容之丰富，为古代本草之冠。且含极丰富之动物、植物、矿物、化学乃至天文、地理、物候等学科知识，故达尔文称其为 "中国古代的百科全书"，近人又称之为博物学巨著。

中国中医科学院图书馆藏

Ben Cao Gang Mu

Ming Dynasty

Ben Cao Gang Mu (Compendium of Materia Medica) was finished in 1578. It is the eighteen years of Ming Dynasty Gengyin (1590) Jinling edition with 52 chapters. This herbal monograph was compiled by Li Shizhen and revised by Li Jianzhong and Li Jianyuan. Chapters 1 and 2 introduce herbal and medicinal theories, and 41 kinds of herbal medicine before the Ming Dynasty. Chapters 3 and 4 are "drugs for hundred of diseases." Chapters 5–52 consist of 1,892 kinds of drugs and 1,109 pictures. With the book *Zheng Lei Ben Cao* (Syndrome of Materia Medica) as the basis, 374 kinds of new drugs were added. This compendium is the integration of herbal medicine of the Ming Dynasty, and the best ancient book in herbalism considering the quantity of drugs and richness of the content. It contains abundant knowledge about animal, vegetable, mineral, chemical and even astronomy, geography, and other disciplines, so Darwin called it "the ancient Chinese encyclopedia," and modern people call it natural history masterpiece.

Preserved in Library of China Academy of Chinese Medical Sciences

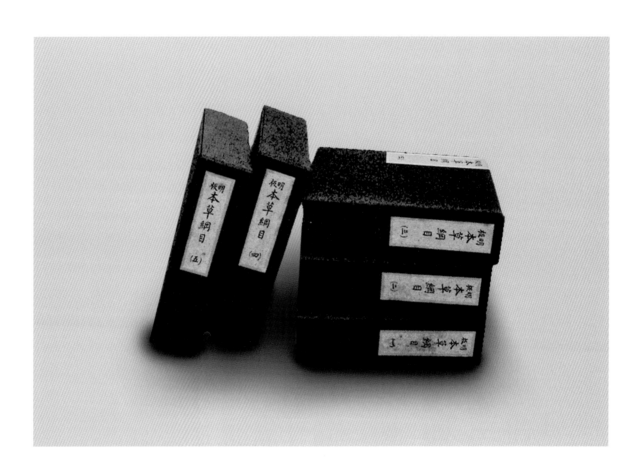

《本草纲目》

明

纵 27.1 厘米，横 17.1 厘米

该藏为明崇祯年（1640）钱蔚起刊本，木雕版线装，共 31 册。书本形，为医籍。《本草纲目》著者为明人李时珍，书凡 52 卷，分水、火、土、金石、草、谷等十六部，共载药 1892 种，是药物学巨著。1578 年成书。保存基本完好，纸张泛黄，边缘有磨损。

中华医学会／上海中医药大学医史博物馆藏

Ben Cao Gang Mu

Ming Dynasty

Vertical Length 27.1 cm/ Horizontal Length 17.1 cm

These preserved collections are Qian Weiqi's edition in the Ming Dynasty (1640). *Ben Cao Gang Mu* (Compendium of Materia Medica), a medical book written by Li Shizhen, has 52 chapters which are divided into 16 parts, namely water, fire, earth, stone, grass, and grain. It introduces a total of 1,892 kinds of drugs. This pharmacological masterpiece was finished in 1578. Woodblock-printed and wire-bound, it is in good condition, expect for the yellow discolouration of the paper and the worn-out edges.

Preserved in Chinese Medical Association/ Museum of Chinese Medicine, Shanghai University of Traditional Chinese Medicine

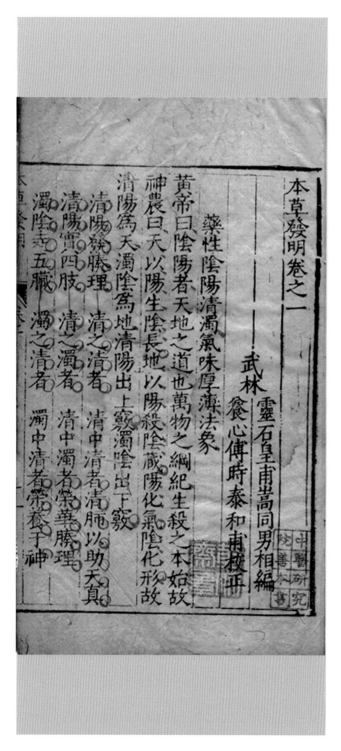

《本草发明》

明

明代木刻本。成书于 1578 年。6 卷。明代皇甫嵩编。本草学专著。卷 1 相当于总论，择要列述金元诸家药理学说。余卷分部议药 600 种，独不取人部之药。各卷置常用药于前，稀用者于后。又设"发明"一项，专于阐述药物主治及配伍要点，简明实用。此本残存卷 1 ～ 4，存药 359 味。

中国中医科学院图书馆藏

Ben Cao Fa Ming

Ming Dynasty

The book is the woodblock edition in the Ming Dynasty. *Ben Cao Fa Ming* (Exposition of Herbs) was compiled by Huangpu Song and finished in 1578. This herbal monograph has 6 chapters. Chapter 1 is equivalent to the pandect, selecting pharmacological doctrine of the Jin and Yuan Dynasties. The rest chapters consist of more than 600 kinds of medicines. In each chapter, commonly used drugs were introduced before the rarely used ones. An item "Fa Ming" was involved in the book to elaborate drug indications and compatibility points, which is concise and practical. This preserved book has only Chapters 1–4, recording 359 medicines.

Preserved in Library of China Academy of Chinese Medical Sciences

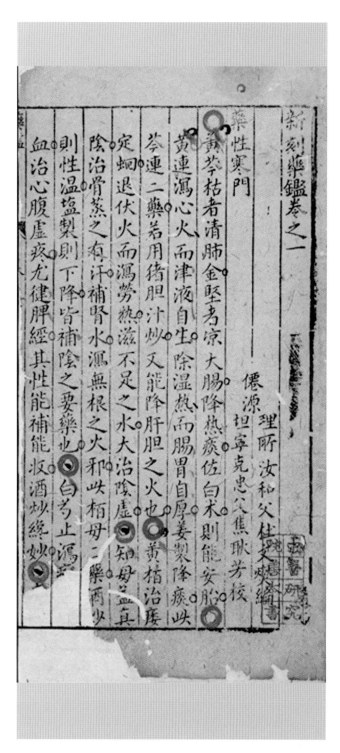

《药鉴》（《新刻药鉴》）

明

明万历二十六年戊戌（1598）木刻本。成书于 1598 年。2 卷。明代杜文燮编，焦耿芳校。本草著作。卷 1 列 27 则专论，主张医者应首察病源，次辨药力；论证则由标本而及经络，审性则由阴阳以及反畏。卷 2 次第叙述 137 种药物之性味及功用，甚便检阅。

中国中医科学院图书馆藏

Yao Jian (*Xin Ke Yao Jian*)

Ming Dynasty

The preserved one is of the woodblock edition in 1598. *Yao Jian* (a medicine handbook) was finished in 1598. This two-chapter book was a herbal masterpiece compiled by Du Wenxie and revised by Jiao Gengfang. Chapter 1 lists 27 monographs advocating that doctors should first examine the sources, and then consider the power of drugs; and analyzing from the incidental and fundamental symptoms to the collateral channels. Chapter 2 introduces the properties, flavors and functions of 137 kinds of drugs in a sequence easy for check.

Preserved in Library of China Academy of Chinese Medical Sciences

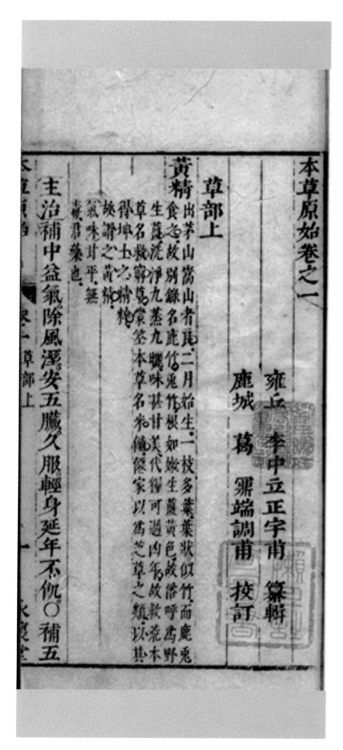

《本草原始》

明

明崇祯十一年戊寅（1638）鹿城木刻本。成书于1612年。12卷。明代李中立纂辑，葛鼎校订。本书共收药452种，附药图379幅。药分草、木、谷、菜、果、石、兽、禽、虫鱼、人10部。每药简述产地、基原形态、性味、主治，后附修治及附方。其临床用药内容多取自《本草纲目》。药图之旁常注明其鉴别要点，此乃该书首创之例；有关药材形态之注文充分汲取了当时药家辨药经验，对药材真伪优劣、道地药材之鉴别甚有裨益，为我国本草史上著名药材学专著。

中国中医科学院图书馆藏

Ben Cao Yuan Shi

Ming Dynasty

The preserved one is of Lucheng woodblock edition in 1638. *Ben Cao Yuan Shi* (Herbal Origin) was finished in 1612. It has 12 chapters, compiled by Li Zhongli and revised by Ge Ding. The book records 452 kinds of drugs, and has 379 drug pictures. Drugs are divided into 10 categories, namely the grass, wood, grain, vegetables, fruit, stone, animals, birds, insects, fish and people. For each drug, the book introduces its original place, original shape, property, flavor, indications, and attached prescriptions. Its clinical contents were mainly retrieved from *Ben Cao Gang Mu* (Compendium of Materia Medica). Next to the diagram of the drug are points to distinguish, which is the innovation of the book; the notes about the form of medicinal drug fully demonstrate the rich herbal experience at that time, which is very beneficial for identifying the quality of medicines. It is a famous monograph on herbal medicines in China.

Preserved in Library of China Academy of Chinese Medical Sciences

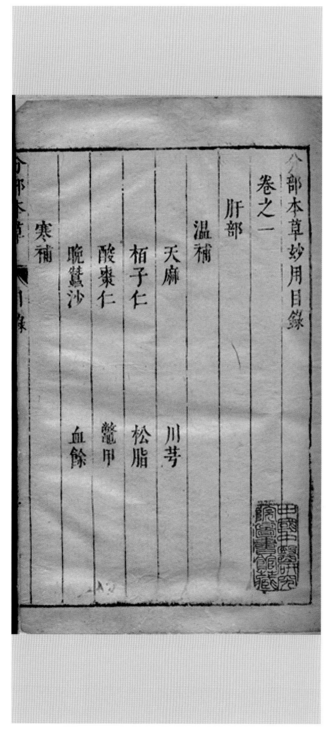

《分部本草妙用》

明

明崇祯木刻本。成书于 1630 年。10 卷。明代顾逢伯撰。本书遵"用药如用兵"之旨，将药物按五脏分部，以仿兵阵之五部；尚有兼经杂药，则按效归类，以仿兵种各有专长。各部类之下，又分温补、寒补、温泻、寒泻、性平 5 种性质归并药物，共叙药 560 余味。各药分别介绍其性味、功效、主治等，述药简明。本书分部新颖，并以药物归经入脏为纲，药效为目，次序井然。

中国中医科学院图书馆藏

Fen Bu Ben Cao Miao Yong

Ming Dynasty

The book is the woodblock edition in the reign of Emperor Chongzhen. *Fen Bu Ben Cao Miao Yong* (Usage of Medicine in Units) was compiled by Gu Fengbo and finished in 1630. It has 10 chapters. Based on the concept that " Using medicine is like deploying military forces", the book divides drugs into five units by internal organs like five units of the army; there are also miscellaneous drugs classified by their effects like different arms of services, such as warm tonification, cold tonification, warm diarrhea, cold diarrhea and mild nature. Concise, innovative and well-organized, this book contains more than 560 kinds of drugs, each being introduced by its property, flavor, effect, indications and so on.

Preserved in Library of China Academy of Chinese Medical Sciences

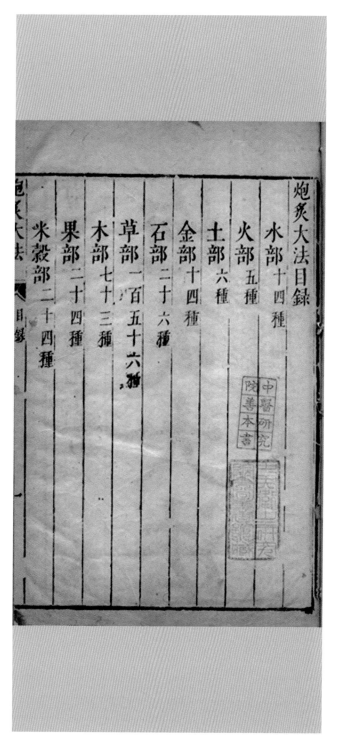

《炮炙大法》

明

明代木刻本。成书于 1622 年。1 卷。明代缪希雍撰，庄继光校。本书系缪氏在其《先醒斋医学广笔记》所载 90 余种炮制品之基础上扩充而成。卷前列"雷公炮制十七法"，继列药物 439 味，分水、火、土、金、石、草、木、果、米谷、菜、人、兽、禽、虫鱼等部。各药条文简要叙其性状鉴别、炮制方法、佐使畏恶等。其中于 172 味药条中引用了《雷公炮炙论》内容，其余则补充了后世炮制法。

中国中医科学院图书馆藏

Pao Zhi Da Fa

Ming Dynasty

The book is the woodblock edition in the Ming Dynasty. *Pao Zhi Da Fa* (Processing of Drugs) was finished in 1622. Woodblock edition, this one-chapter book was compiled by Miao Xiyong and proofread by Zhuang Jiguang. Miao completed this book on the basis of more than 90 kinds of processed products recorded in another medical book, *Xian Xing Zhai Yi Xue Guang Bi Ji*. The chapter started with "Seventeen Methods for Concocting Drugs" followed by 439 drugs, which are classified into units like water, fire, earth, metal, stone, grass, wood, fruit, grain, vegetables, people, animals, birds, insects, fish, and so on. Each entry briefly introduces how to identify and process the drugs. Contents of 172 drugs were cited from *Lei Gong Pao Zhi Lun* (Leigong Treatise on Processing), with the rest being the new supplement.

Preserved in Library of China Academy of Chinese Medical Sciences

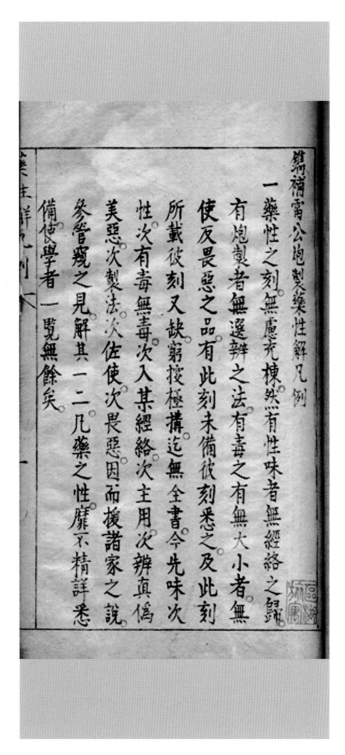

《雷公炮制药性解》

明

明天启二年壬戌（1622）木刻本。成书于
1622年。6卷。明代李中梓编辑，钱允治订正。
本书以李中梓之《药性解》（2卷）为本，
增入《雷公炮炙论》135条条文于相应药条
之后而成。其内容仍以临证用药为主，非为
炮制专书。全书收药323味，分金石、果、
谷、草、木、菜、人、禽兽、虫鱼9部。"药
性解"部分各药简述性味、归经、功治，又
附作者按语，注解药性及提示用药要点，简
洁明了，常出新见。

中国中医科学院图书馆藏

Lei Gong Pao Zhi Yao Xing Jie (Engraved Supplement Edition)

Ming Dynasty

The book is the woodblock edition in 1622. The book *Lei Gong Pao Zhi Yao Xing Jie* (Herbal Solution of Lei Gong Treatise on Processing) was finished in 1622. The six-chapter book was compiled by Li Zhongzi and proofread by Qian Yunzhi. On the basis of Li Zhongzi's book *Yao Xing Jie* (Herbal Solution) (2 chapters), this book adds 135 items from *Lei Gong Pao Zhi Lun* (Lei Gong Treatise on Processing). Its content is still dominated by clinical medicine, not only for processing products. The book records 323 drugs and is divided into 9 sections, namely stone, fruit, grain, grass, wood, food, people, animals, as well as insects and fish. "Herbal Solution" section gives a brief introduction to the property, flavor, channel tropism, and effect of each drug, with authors' notes, comments and tips of herbal medication, which is concise and original.

Preserved in Library of China Academy of Chinese Medical Sciences

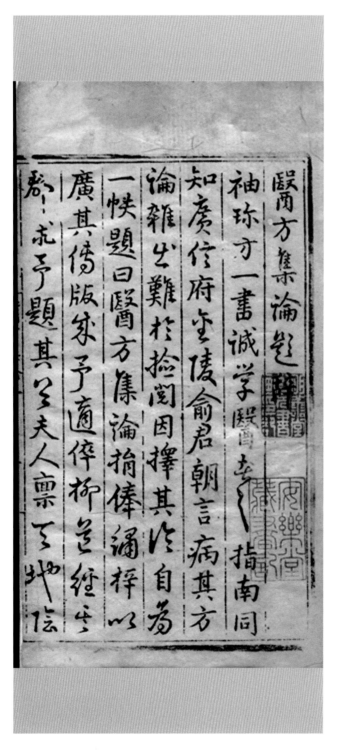

《医方集论》

明

明弘治六年癸丑（1493）木刻本。成书于1493 年。不分卷。明代俞朝言撰。中医证候学专著。首论风、寒、暑、湿四气致病之型证特点，次叙伤寒、疟、痢、呕吐、泄泻、霍乱、秘结、咳嗽等内、外、妇、儿各科证候 50 余种，每类证候述其病因病机、脉证、治则，或述分类，所论简明扼要，持论中正。

中国中医科学院图书馆藏

Yi Fang Ji Lun

Ming Dynasty

The book is the woodblock edition in 1493. *Yi Fang Ji Lun* (A Collection of Prescriptions) was written by Yu Zhaoyan and finished in 1493. It was not divided into chapters. This symptomatology monograph of traditional Chinese medicine first states features of diseases caused by wind, cold, heat, and wet, and then describes 50 syndromes from internal medicine, surgery, gynecology and pediatrics, consisting of typhoid fever, malaria, dysentery, vomiting, diarrhea, cholera, constipation and cough. Each syndrome is described from its pathogenesis, pulse and signs, treatment, or classification, which is concise and objective.

Preserved in Library of China Academy of Chinese Medical Sciences

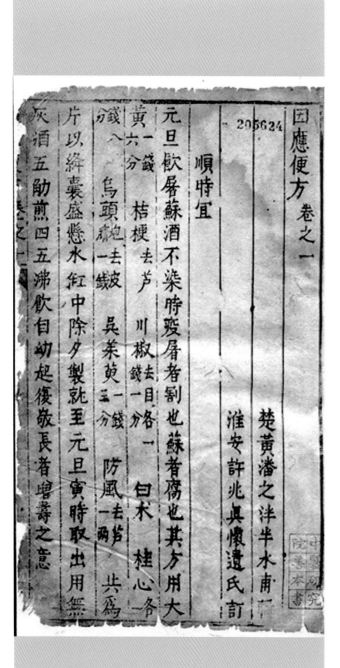

因應便方 卷之一

順時宜

楚黃潘之泮半水甫□
淮安許兆真懷遠氏訂

元旦飲屠蘇酒不染時疫屠者割也蘇者腐也其方用大

黃一錢　桔梗去芦　川椒錢去目各一分

防風去芦

白术桂心各

吳茱萸三分

烏頭炮去皮一錢

右以絳囊盛懸水缸中除夕製就至元旦寅時取出用無

灰酒五勺煎四五沸飲自幼起復敬長者增壽之意

《因应便方》

明

明刻本。成书于 1522 年。2 卷。明代潘之泮辑，许兆真订。中医方书著作。首述用药顺时宜、卫生却病等，以下录卷君长命丹、不老丹、延命固本丹等各种用方 500 余首。其卷二之"神授秘诀歌"，用歌诀体叙内、外、妇、儿科等常见病症及其验方 60 余首。该书之主要特点是所载之方多不见于其他方书，而为本书独存。

中国中医科学院图书馆藏

Yin Ying Bian Fang

Ming Dynasty

The book is the block-printed edition in the Ming Dynasty. *Yin Ying Bian Fang* (Prescriptions for Convenience) was finished in 1522. The book has 2 chapters. It was compiled by Pan Zhipan and was proofread by Xu Zhaozhen in the Ming Dynasty. In the first chapter of this traditional Chinese medical prescription book, it describes how to use medicine in accordance with time, including more than 500 prescriptions. The second chapter describes common diseases such as internal, surgical, gynecological and pediatric diseases in style of rhymes and records over 60 prescriptions. The main characteristic of this book is the exclusive prescriptions in it, which are not seen in other books.

Preserved in Library of China Academy of Chinese Medical Sciences

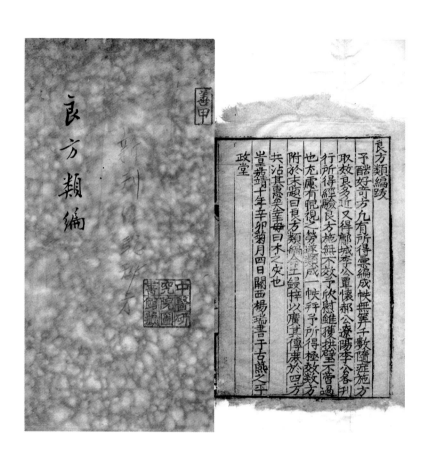

《良方类编》

明

平政堂刊本，明嘉靖十年辛卯（1531）古燕木刻本。 成书于 1531 年。53 页。本书系医方丛书，合刊方书 3 种：《新刊经验秘方》由明代张子麒辑，收方 28 首，其目录每方下即标明药味之数；《方外奇方》撰人不详，收方 23 首，每方叙制法、服法尤详；《经验药方》系明代李文敏等辑，收方 13 首，末附杨氏新辑七圣万灵丹等 5 方，收方以单验秘方为主。

中国中医科学院图书馆藏

Liang Fang Lei Bian

Ming Dynasty

The preserved one was of Ping Zheng Tang publication and Gu Yan woodblock edition in 1531. *Liang Fang Lei Bian* (Classification of Effective Prescriptions) was finished in 1531. This medical prescription collection has 53 pages and consists of three parts: *Xin Kan Jing Yan Mi Fang* (New Edition of Experienced Secrete Prescriptions) compiled by Zhang Ziqi in the Ming Dynasty, recording 28 prescriptions, with the number of medicines marked under each prescription in the catalogue. *Fang Wai Qi Fang* (Odd-ingredient Prescriptions), the editor of which is unknown, recorded 23 prescriptions, each with detailed processing method and instructions. *Jing Yan Yao Fang* (Experienced Secrete Prescriptions) was compiled by Li Wenmin and others in the Ming Dynasty, recording 13 prescriptions. In the end there are five prescriptions compiled by Yang. The prescriptions recorded in this book are mainly secret recipes.

Preserved in Library of China Academy of Chinese Medical Sciences

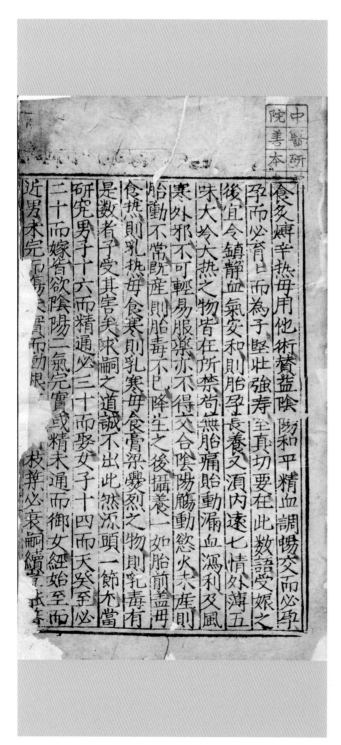

《万氏积善堂集验方》

明

明刻本。成书于 1536 年。3 卷。明代鹿园居士辑。本书卷上"广嗣要语"，收男女服药论、调元、调经、安胎等简短医论，并金锁思仙丹、五子衍宗丸等嗣育方近 50 首；卷中录滋补方 50 首，并附元代王隐君"论童壮""论衰老"两篇医论；卷下杂录各科验方 60 余首。

中国中医科学院图书馆藏

Wan Shi Ji Shan Tang Ji Yan Fang

Ming Dynasty

The book is the block-printed edition in the Ming Dynasty. The book *Wan Shi Ji Shan Tang Ji Yan Fang* (Collected Prescription of Wan's Ji Shan Tang) is a three-chapter book compiled by Luyuan Jushi and finished in 1536. Chapter I "Guang Si Yao Yu" (Tips to Having More Children), exposes brief medical theories on medications for men and women, regulation of vigour and menstruation, miscarriage prevention and so on. Chapter I has nearly 50 parenting prescriptions. Chapter Ⅱ has 50 nourishing prescriptions and two medical treatises "On Youth" and "On Aging" written by Wang Yinjun of the Yuan Dynasty. Chapter Ⅲ has a miscellany of more than 60 various prescriptions.

Preserved in Library of China Academy of Chinese Medical Sciences

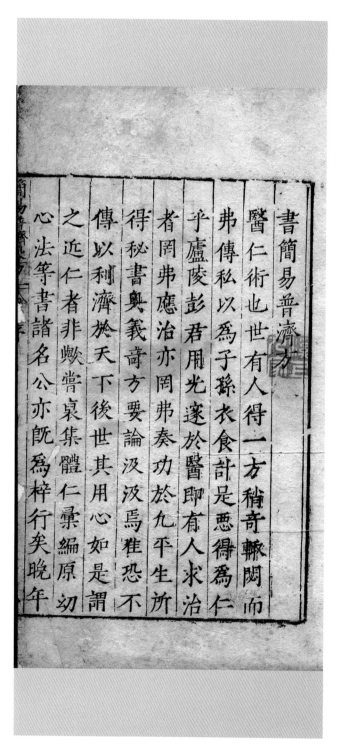

《简易普济良方》

明

明嘉靖四十年辛酉（1561）木刻本。成书
于1561年。6卷。明代彭用光编集。方书。
本书分中风、诸风、伤寒、辟瘟疫、风湿、
痰等门，分门汇辑历代医籍及民间单验方。
卷5录"痈疽神妙灸经"，附图16幅，各
具痈疽之状、灸治穴位。

中国中医科学院图书馆藏

Jian Yi Pu Ji Liang Fang

Ming Dynasty

The preserved one is of the woodblock edition in 1561. *Jian Yi Pu Ji Liang Fang* (Simple Prescriptions for Common Disease) was compiled by Peng Yongguang and finished in 1561. The six-chapter book contains prescriptions from medical classics as well as folk prescriptions in past dynasties under categories like stroke, various wind pathogens, exogenous febrile disease, pestilence, rheumatism, phlegm and so on. In the 5th chapter, "Yong Ju Shen Miao Jiu Jing" (treatment of ulcer by moxibustion) has 16 attached pictures for signs of different ulcers and acupuncture points of moxibustion.

Preserved in Library of China Academy of Chinese Medical Sciences

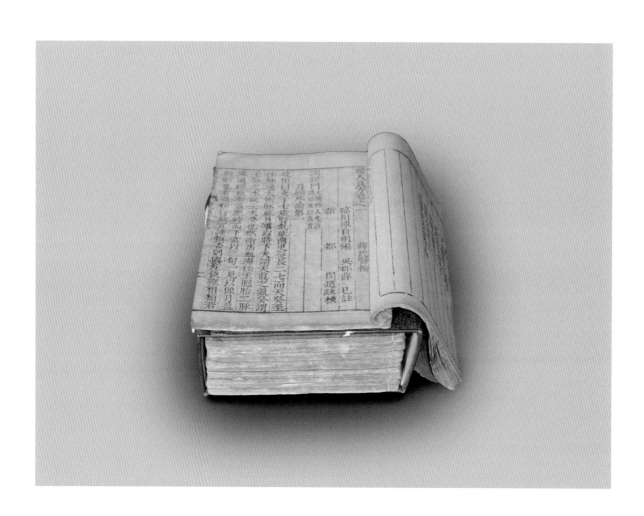

《**妇人大全良方**》

明

嘉靖二十六年（1547）刻本。宋代陈自明（良甫）撰。1 函 12 册。陕西中医药大学图书馆调拨。

陕西医史博物馆藏

Fu Ren Da Quan Liang Fang

Ming Dynasty

The book is the block-printed edition in 1547.

Fu Ren Da Quan Liang Fang (a medical book on gynaecology and obstetrics) was written from Chen Ziming (Liangfu) in the Song Dynasty and finished in 1547. The preserved collection has 12 volumes in 1 case. It was allocated from the Library of Shaanxi University of Chinese Medicine.

Preserved in Shaanxi Museum of Medical History

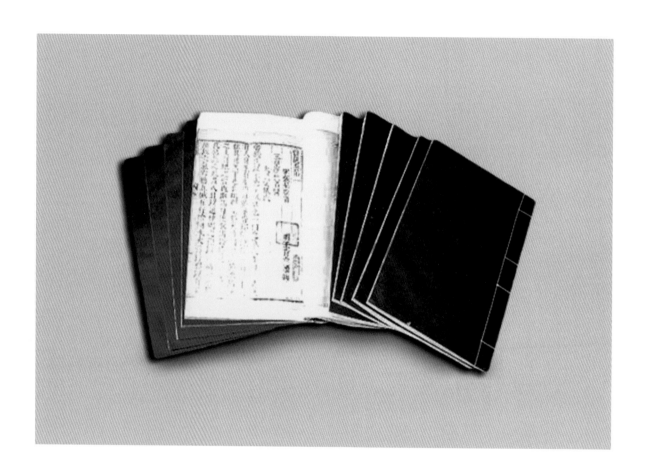

《医说》书影

明

明刻本。宋代张杲原著。王肯堂续辑。作者张杲，字季明，宋代新安（今安徽歙县）人，具体生卒年代无考，大约生活在南宋初期。张杲的医术师其父张彦仁，彦仁师其父张子发，子发师其兄张子充，子充则师于庞安时，所谓三世之医也。张杲欲博观远望，弘扬医道，凡书之有涉于医者，必记之，辑成一部，名之曰《医说》。《医说》10卷，分三皇历代名医、医书、本草、针灸等49门，凡925条。全书引用宋代及宋以前文史医药典籍130余种之多，是一部内容丰富的医学文献资料。

南京中医药大学图书馆藏

Book Photograph of *Yi Shuo*

Ming Dynasty

The preserved collection is the block-printed edition of the Ming Dynasty. It was originally authored by Zhang Gao in the Song Dynasty and later supplemented by Wang Kentang in the Ming Dynasty. Zhang Gao, style name Jiming, was born in Xin'an (now in Shexian County, Anhui Province). The date of his birth and death is unknown, but he lived approximately in the early Southern Song Dynasty. His family had practiced medicine for three generations since Zhang Gao's grandfather's elder brother learnt medicine from Pang Anshi, a famous doctor in the Northern Song Dynasty, and then the profession was passed down successively through his grandfather Zhang Zifa, his father Zhang Yanren, and to him at last. Zhang Gao read extensively, had visionary thoughts, and carried forward medical science. He collected everything about medicine ever recorded in books and compiled them into the ten-chapter book Yi Shuo, which covers 925 items in 49 categories, including famous doctors in the previous dynasties, medical books, medical herbs, and acupuncture and moxibustion. The book quoted more than 130 classics about literature, history and medicine of the Song and the previous dynasties, making it a valuable medical document with abundant information.

Preserved in Library of Nanjing University of Chinese Medicine

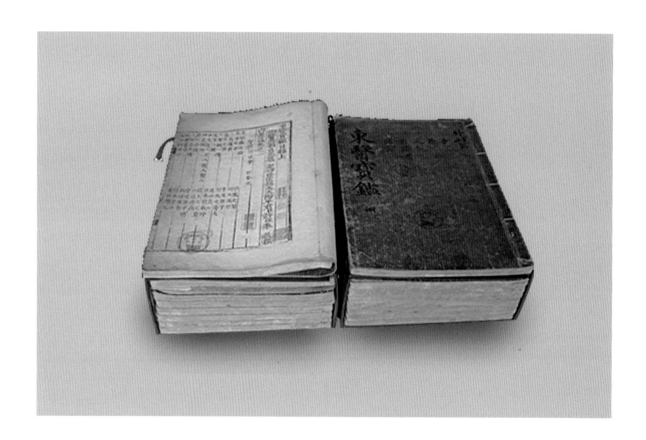

《东医宝鉴》

明

旧刻本。朝鲜许浚等著，3 函 25 册。1613 年内医院初刻本，现藏韩国首尔大学图书馆奎章阁。中国最早的刻本是中国中医科学院图书馆藏乾隆二十八年癸未（1763）壁鱼堂沃根园刻本。保存完整。陕西中医药大学图书馆调拨。

陕西医史博物馆藏

Dong Yi Bao Jian

Ming Dynasty

Written by Xu Jun and others in Korea, the book is the old block-printed edition with 25 volumes in 3 cases. The first block-printed edition of *Dong Yi Bao Jian* by Korean Royal Hospital in 1613 is now preserved in Kyujanggak Institute of Seoul National University Library. The earliest block-printed edition in China was made by Wogenyuan of Bi Yu Tang bookstore in 1763, which is now preserved in Library of China Academy of Chinese Medical Sciences in Beijing. It is well preserved and was allocated from the Library of Shaanxi University of Chinese Medicine.

Preserved in Shaanxi Museum of Medical History

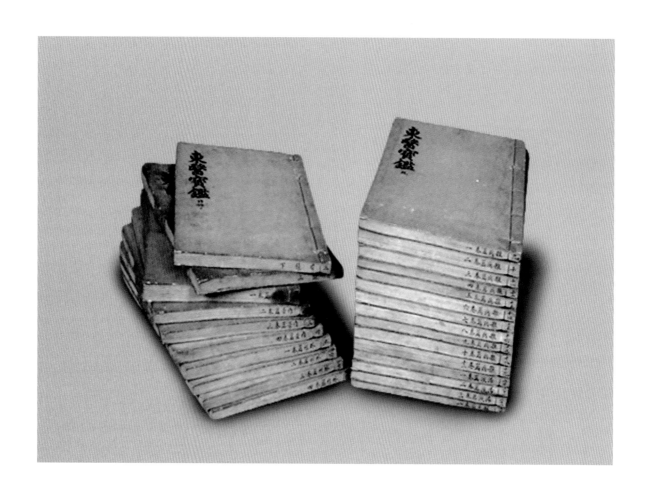

《东医宝鉴》

明

纵 17 厘米，横 11.3 厘米

明万历医籍，书本形。《东医宝鉴》，朝鲜医家许浚等著。全书 23 卷，共 25 册。版本待考。保存基本完整，纸张泛黄，局部磨损。

中华医学会 / 上海中医药大学医史博物馆藏

Dong Yi Bao Jian

Ming Dynasty

Vertical Length17cm/ Horizontal Length 11.3 cm

Dong Yi Bao Jian is a book series about medical knowledge in East Asia, written by Korean medical scientist Xu Jun and others in the reign of Emperor Wanli of the Ming Dynasty. The preserved collection has 23 chapters and 25 volumes, but the edition needs to be verified. These books are basically in complete condition, with yellow discolouration of the paper and the worn-out edges.

Preserved in Chinese Medical Association/ Museum of Chinese Medicine, Shanghai University of Traditional Chinese Medicine

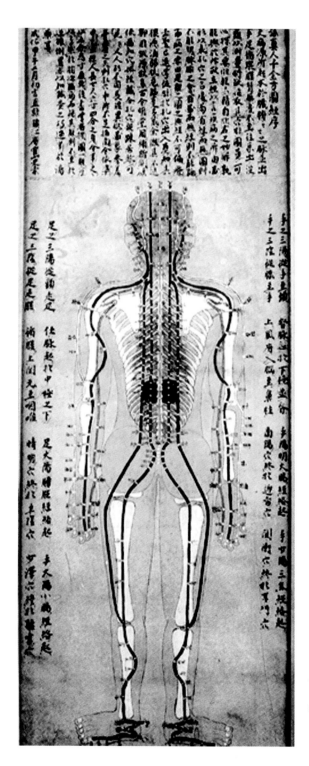

《针灸明堂图》

明

背面经穴图。上有史素于明成化甲午年（1474）

撰书之"孙真人千金方图经序"。

荷兰国立民族学博物馆藏

Zhen Jiu Ming Tang Tu

Ming Dynasty

This picture is a figure of channels and acupuncture points of the human back. There are also the Chinese characters reading "Sun Zhen Ren Qian Jin Fang Tu Jing Xu" (the preface of a Chinese medical prescription book) written by Shi Su in 1474.

Preserved in National Museum of Ethnology

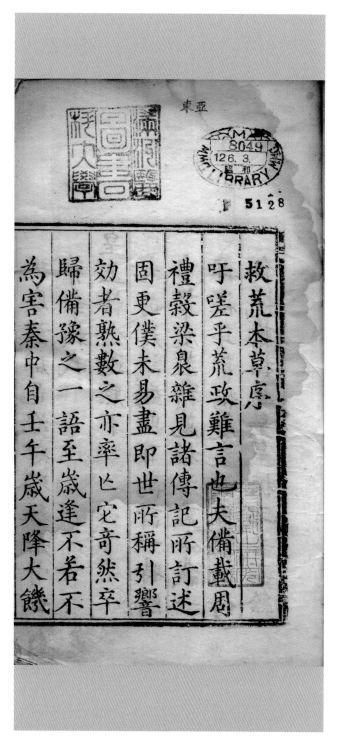

《救荒本草》

明

明万历十四年丙戌（1586）木刻本。成书于
1406 年。2 卷。明代朱橚撰。本书收可食
植物 414 种，其中此书新增者 276 种，分草、
木、米、谷、菜、果 6 部。各物简述其产地、
形态、性味、良毒及烹调食用方法，内容确
切实用。每物一图，图文并茂。其图均来自
于实物写生，甚为精致。本书为我国 15 世
纪的一部著名的植物学图谱，对后世农学、
植物学及医药学发展均有重要影响。该书流
传到日本后，对其农学、植物学发展亦有很
大促进，并产生了众多后续性著作。

中国中医科学院图书馆藏

Jiu Huang Ben Cao

Ming Dynasty

The preserved one is block-printed edition in 1586. *Jiu Huang Ben Cao* (Herbal for Relief of Famines) was written by Zhu Su in the Ming Dynasty and finished in 1406. The two-chapter book records 414 edible plants (among which 276 were newly added in this book) in 6 sections: grass, wood, rice, grain, vegetables and fruits. For each object, there are brief descriptions of its producing area, appearance, property and flavor, benignancy or toxicity and the way of cooking, and attached with an exquisite drawing from nature. This book is an important botanical atlas in the 15th century and had profound influence on the later development of agronomy, botany, medicine and pharmacology. After it was spread to Japan, it had greatly promoted the development of the agronomy and botany there, and led to many subsequent works.

Preserved in Library of China Academy of Chinese Medical Sciences

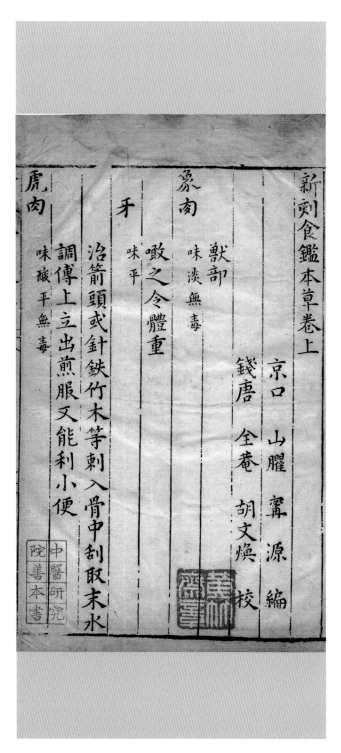

《食鉴本草》（《新刻食鉴本草》）

明

明万历二十年壬辰（1592）虎林木刻本。成书于1566年。明代宁源编，胡文焕校。本书收兽、禽、虫、果等可食之品百余种，简述其性味功治，并附前人论说及方剂，间有己意。曾为《本草纲目》所引，但李时珍评谓："略载数语，无所发明。"此本仅残存卷上。

中国中医科学院图书馆藏

Shi Jian Ben Cao (New Edition)

Ming Dynasty

The book is the Hulin woodblock edition in 1592. *Shi Jian Ben Cao* (Dietary Materia Medica) was compiled by Ning Yuan (Ming Dynasty), proofread by Hu Wenhuan (Ming Dynasty) and finished in 1566. This book contains more than one hundred edible species like beasts, birds, insects and fruits, with brief descriptions of their property, flavor and curative effect, including the relevant exposition and prescriptions from the previous books or the author's personal comments. This book was once quoted by *Ben Cao Gang Mu* (Compendium of Materia Medica), but was commented by its author,Li Shizhen, as "too brief to have innovation". There remains only Chapter I in the preserved collection.

Preserved in Library of China Academy of Chinese Medical Sciences

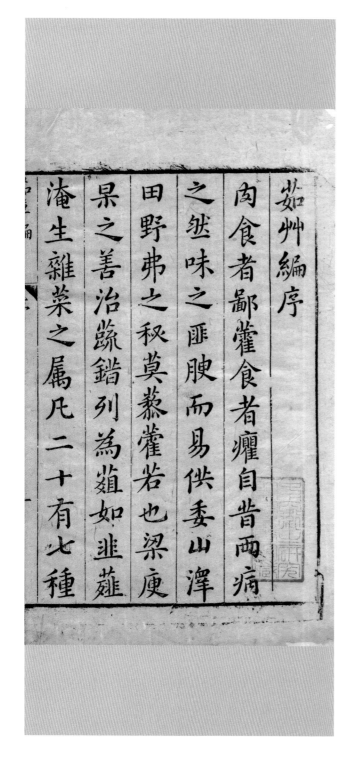

《茹草编》

明

明万历二十五年丁酉（1597）金陵木刻本。
成书于1582年。4卷。明代周履靖著，周
绍濂校。本书共集录102种可食野生植物资
料。卷1首载《茹草解》《飡英歌》，次载
草物50种。每物一图一诗，兼注食用方法。
诗文典雅悠闲，图形较精，多由写生绘成。
卷3、4为《茹草纪言》，系汇集前人书中
有关可食野生植物之说。

中国中医科学院图书馆藏

Ru Cao Bian

Ming Dynasty

The book is the Jinling woodblock edition in 1597. *Ru Cao Bian* (A Book about Materials of Edible Wild Plants) was written by Zhou Lüjing (Ming Dynasty), proofread by Zhou Shaolian (Ming Dynasty) and finished in 1582. The four-chapter book records 102 edible wild plants. Chapter I contains *Ru Cao Jie* and *Xiang Ying Ge* (records of plants) at the beginning, followed by 50 herbal species. Every object is attached with a picture and a poem, and is given a clear indication of its edible methods. The poems are refined and relaxing, while the pictures, made according to paint of life, are quite exquisite. The 3rd and 4th chapters are *Ru Cao Ji Yan*, recording the previous theories of edible wild plants.

Preserved in Library of China Academy of Chinese Medical Sciences

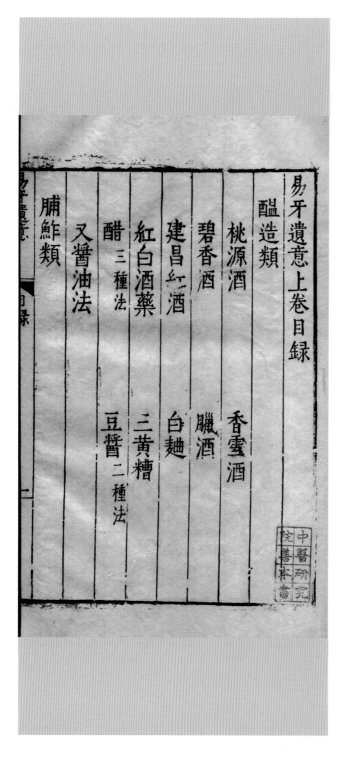

《易牙遗意》

明

明万历木刻本。成书于 1582 年。2 卷。明代韩奕编，周履靖校。本书为烹饪著作，分酿造、脯脂、蔬菜、炉造、糕饵、汤饼、斋食、果实、诸汤、诸茶、食药等类，述食品143种，介绍其制作方法，其中亦有与医药相关之内容。书末附宋代朱翼中所著之《酒经》。

中国中医科学院图书馆藏

Yi Ya Yi Yi

Ming Dynasty

The book is the woodblock edition in the regin of Emperor Wanli of the Ming Dynasty. *Yi Ya Yi Yi* (A Book of Cooking and Medical Knowledge) was compiled by Han Yi of the Ming Dynasty, proofread by Zhou Lüjing of the Ming Dynasty and finished in 1582. The two-chapter book is a masterpiece on cooking, including 143 kinds of food in categories like brewed, preserved, steamed and stoved food, as well as vegetables, cakes, vegetarian food, fruits, soups, tea and edible medicine. Cooking methods of the food and relevant medical knowledge were introduced. At the end of the book, *Jiu Jing* (A Book on Wine-making Technology) written by Zhu Yizhong in the Song Dynasty is attached.

Preserved in Library of China Academy of Chinese Medical Sciences

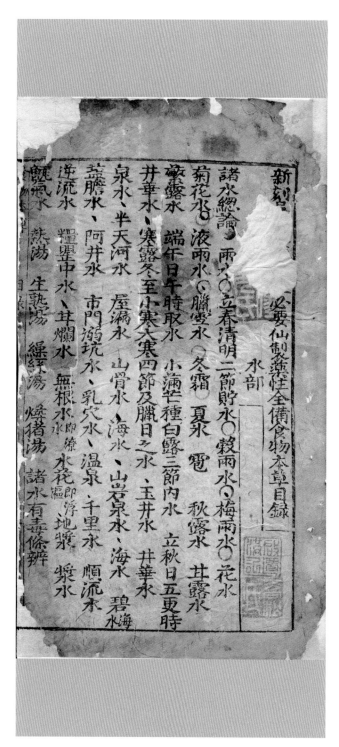

《新刻吴氏家传养生必要仙制药性全备食物本草》

明

明代木刻本。成书于 1593 年。4 卷。明代吴文炳汇编。本草学专著。本书共收食品 459 种，并附汤、酒、粥百余种，诸品分水、五谷、菜、果、兽、禽、虫、鱼数类。每品均叙述产地、形态、性味、功用、宜忌等，内容多系摘引诸家本草。

中国中医科学院图书馆藏

New Edition of Herbal Collection by Wu's Family

Ming Dynasty

The book is the woodblock edition in the Ming Dynasty. This four-chapter agrostology monograph was compiled by Wu Wenbing (Ming Dynasty) and finished in 1593. It contains 459 kinds of food, as well as more than a hundred kinds of soup, wines and porridge, under the categories of water, grains, vegetables, fruits, beasts, birds, insects, fish and so on. Each food is described in detail with its place of production, form, property and flavor, effect, compatibility and incompatibility. These contents were mostly extracted from different herbal classics.

 Preserved in Library of China Academy of Chinese Medical Sciences

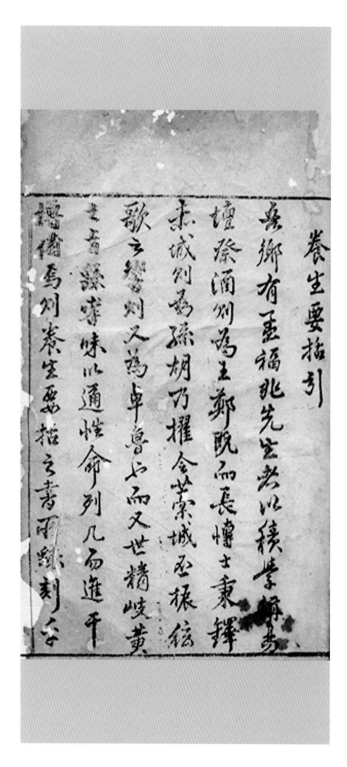

《养生要括》

明

明崇祯七年甲戌（1634）刻本。成书于
1634 年。1 卷。明代孟笨编。本草类著作。
摘取《本草纲目》中 250 种饮食物的有关
资料编成。各物简述其性味主治，偶加自注，
但少发挥。

中国中医科学院图书馆藏

Yang Sheng Yao Kuo

Ming Dynasty

The book is the block-printed edition in 1634.
Yang Sheng Yao Kuo (A Monograph of Food
and Herbal Medicine) was written by Meng Ben
(Ming Dynasty) and finished in 1634. This one-
chapter book records 250 kinds of food and drink
extracted from *Ben Cao Gang Mu* (Compendium
of Materia Medica). The author briefly described
the property, flavor and function of each item
with some occasional footnotes.

Preserved in Library of China Academy of Chinese
Medical Sciences

祝允明《饭苓赋》轴

明

纵 142.8 厘米，横 27.9 厘米

进士刘时君作。墨迹，笔法精谨，墨方圆变化多样，字体清劲。

故宫博物院藏

Scroll of *Fan Ling Fu* by Zhu Yunming

Ming Dynasty

Vertical Length 142.8 cm/ Horizontal Length 27.9 cm

This scroll of calligraphy work was written in running hand and regular script with black ink. Its technique is exquisite and cautious with various artistic and powerful styles.

Preserved in The Palace Museum

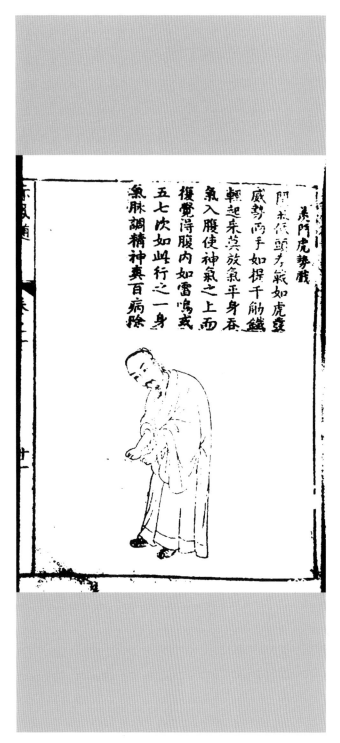

《五禽戏图》

明

长 27.6 厘米，宽 17.3 厘米

该藏为明代周履靖《赤凤髓》一书，明万历刻本（1579）中之五禽戏图。五禽戏是东汉医家华佗发明的模仿熊、鹿、虎、猿和鸟五种动物运动的体育医疗术，认为体有不快，作一禽之戏则舒。即人体须得劳动，动摇则谷气得消，血脉流通，病不得生。此为"羡门虎势戏"图。1960 年入藏。保存基本完好。

中华医学会／上海中医药大学医史博物馆藏

Wu Qin Xi Tu

Ming Dynasty

Length 27.6 cm/ Width 17.3 cm

Wu Qin Xi Tu (Figure of Medical Exercises Imitating Movements of Five Animals) belongs to medical classics. The preserved one is the block-printed edition(1579) of *Chi Feng Sui* (A Medical Book of A System of Deep Breathing Exercises) written by Zhou Lüjing. Wu Qin Xi, an exercise created by medical scientist Hua Tuo in the Eastern Han Dynasty, is an athletic medical treatment by the movements imitating bear, deer, tiger, ape and bird. Hua Tuo believed that the discomfort of the body could be cured by medical exercises imitating movements of animals. By doing so, the essence derived from food will be digested, the blood and "Qi" in the vessel will be unblocked and people will not get sick. The picture shows a figure called "Xian Men Hu Shi Xi" (the exercise imitating the movement of tiger). It was collected in 1960 and is basically preserved in good condition.

Preserved in Chinese Medical Association/ Museum of Chinese Medicine, Shanghai University of Traditional Chinese Medicine

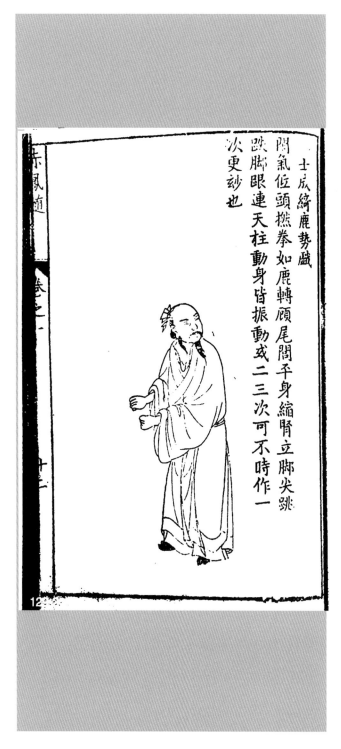

士成绮鹿势戏

闭气低头攒拳如鹿转顾尾闾平身缩肾立脚尖跳

跌脚跟连天柱动身皆振动或二三次可不时作一

次更妙也

《五禽戏图》

明

长 27.6 厘米，宽 17.3 厘米

该藏为明代周履靖《赤凤髓》一书，明万历
刻本（1579）中之五禽戏图。此为"士成绮
鹿势戏"图。1960 年入藏。保存基本完好。

中华医学会／上海中医药大学医史博物馆藏

Wu Qin Xi Tu

Ming Dynasty

Length 27.6 cm/ Width 17.3 cm

Wu Qin Xi Tu (Figures of Medical Exercises Imitating Movements of Five Animals) belongs to medical classics. The preserved one is the block-printed edition (1579) of *Chi Feng Sui* (A Medical Book of A System of Deep Breathing Exercises) written by Zhou Lüjing. This is a figure called "Shi Cheng Qi Lu Shi Xi" (the exercise imitating the movement of deer). It was collected in 1960 and is basically preserved in good condition.

Preserved in Chinese Medical Association/ Museum of Chinese Medicine, Shanghai University of Traditional Chinese Medicine

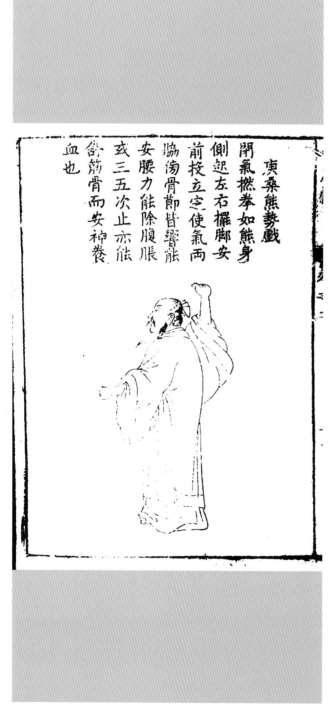

《五禽戏图》

明

长 27.6 厘米，宽 17.3 厘米

该藏为明代周履靖《赤凤髓》一书，明万历

刻本（1579）中之五禽戏图。此为"庚桑熊

势戏"图。1960 年入藏。保存基本完好。

中华医学会/上海中医药大学医史博物馆藏

Wu Qin Xi Tu

Ming Dynasty

Length 27.6 cm/ Width 17.3 cm

Wu Qin Xi Tu (Figures of Medical Exercises Imitating Movements of Five Animals) belongs to medical classics. The preserved one is the block-printed edition (1579) of *Chi Feng Sui* (A Medical Book of A System of Deep Breathing Exercises) written by Zhou Lüjing. This is a figure called "Geng Sang Xiong Shi Xi" (the exercise imitating the movement of bear). It was collected in 1960 and is basically preserved in good condition.

Preserved in Chinese Medical Association/ Museum of Chinese Medicine, Shanghai University of Traditional Chinese Medicine

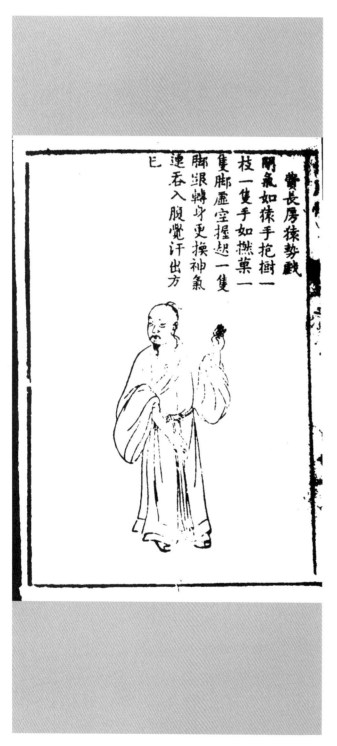

《五禽戏图》

明

长 27.6 厘米，宽 17.3 厘米

该藏为明代周履靖《赤凤髓》一书，明万历刻本（1579）中之五禽戏图。此为"费长房猿势戏"图。1960 年入藏。保存基本完好。

中华医学会 / 上海中医药大学医史博物馆藏

Wu Qin Xi Tu

Ming Dynasty

Length 27.6 cm/ Width 17.3 cm

Wu Qin Xi Tu (Figures of Medical Exercises Imitating Movements of Five Animals) belongs to medical classics. The preserved one is the block-printed edition (1579) of *Chi Feng Sui* (A Medical Book of A System of Deep Breathing Exercises) written by Zhou Lüjing. This is a figure called "Fei Zhang Fang Yuan Shi Xi" (the exercise imitating the movement of ape). It was collected in 1960 and is basically preserved in good condition.

Preserved in Chinese Medical Association/ Museum of Chinese Medicine, Shanghai University of Traditional Chinese Medicine

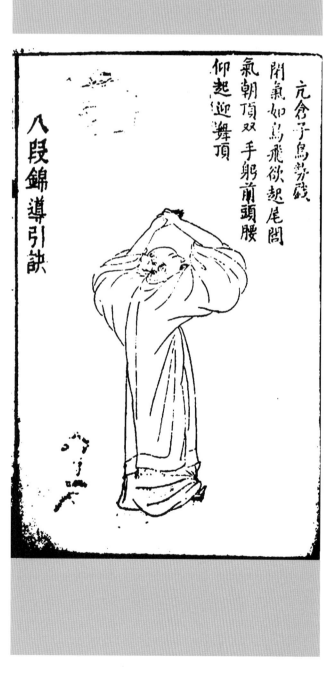

《五禽戏图》

明

长 27.6 厘米，宽 17.3 厘米

该藏为明代周履靖《赤凤髓》一书，明万历
刻本（1579）中之五禽戏图。此为"亢仓子
鸟势戏"图。1960 年入藏。保存基本完好。

中华医学会／上海中医药大学医史博物馆藏

Wu Qin Xi Tu

Ming Dynasty

Length 27.6 cm/ Width 17.3 cm

Wu Qin Xi Tu (Figures of Medical Exercises Imitating Movements of Five Animals) belongs to medical classics. The preserved one is the block-printed edition (1579) of *Chi Feng Sui* (A Medical Book of A System of Deep Breathing Exercises) written by Zhou Lüjing. This is a figure called "Kang Cang Zi Niao Shi Xi" (the exercise imitating the movement of bird). It was collected in 1960 and is basically preserved in good condition.

Preserved in Chinese Medical Association/ Museum of Chinese Medicine, Shanghai University of Traditional Chinese Medicine

丸經集叙

捶丸古戰國之遺策也粤若稽古莊子之書昔
者楚莊王偃兵宋都得市南勇士熊宜僚者工
於九上衆稱之以當五百人乗以劒而不動捶
九九於千一軍停戰而觀之莊王免於敵而覇
降世尚習益聞而知之未造其理也至宋徽宗
金章宗皆愛捶丸盛以錦囊擊以綵棒碾玉綴
頂飾金緑邊深求古人之遺製而益致其精也
且夫飽食終日無所用心不有博弈者乎爲之
猶賢乎巳而聖人稱之方今天下隆平邊陲寧

佚名《丸经》书影

明

边框：宽 13 厘米，高 17 厘米

该书共 2 卷，32 章。关于当时流行的捶丸
活动的场地、用具、竞赛方式、竞赛人数以
及竞赛规则等，此书均作了专门、详细的记
述，是关于古代捶丸活动的重要著述。此书
收录于明嘉靖年间（1522—1566）刻本《小
十三经》的第四册。

中国国家图书馆藏

Book Photograph of *Wan Jing* (Anonymous)

Ming Dynasty

Frame: Width 13 cm/ Height 17 cm

Wan Jing is an important book about an ancient game "Chui Wan" (to strike the ball with a stick). With 2 chapters and 32 chapters, it makes a special and detailed record of the exercise yard, equipment, way of competition, number of players, rules of the game, etc. The preserved collection was from Book Ⅳ of *Xiao Shi San Jing* (the Minor Thirteen Confucian Classics) with the edition during the reign of Emperor Jiajing (1522–1566) of the Ming Dynasty.

Preserved in National Library of China

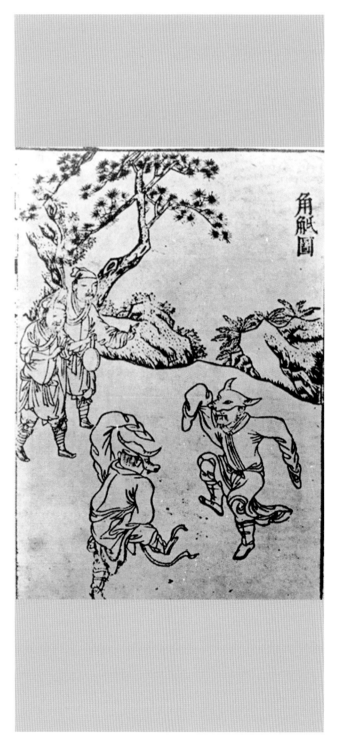

《三才图会·角抵图》

明

万历三十七年刊本。106卷，明代王圻、王思义编著。此《角抵图》为其中插图之一，描写了两位头戴牛头假面的武士正在进行摔跤的情景。

中国国家图书馆藏

San Cai Tu Hui- Jiao Di Tu

Ming Dynasty

The preserved edition was published in 1609.
San Cai Tu Hui (an illustrated ancient Chinese encyclopedia about everything in sky, earth and human world) is composed of 106 chapters and was compiled by Wang Qi and Wang Siyi in the Ming Dynasty. *Jiao Di Tu* (Wrestling Painting) is one of the insets of this book, which describes two warriors wrestling with ox-head masks.

Preserved in National Library of China

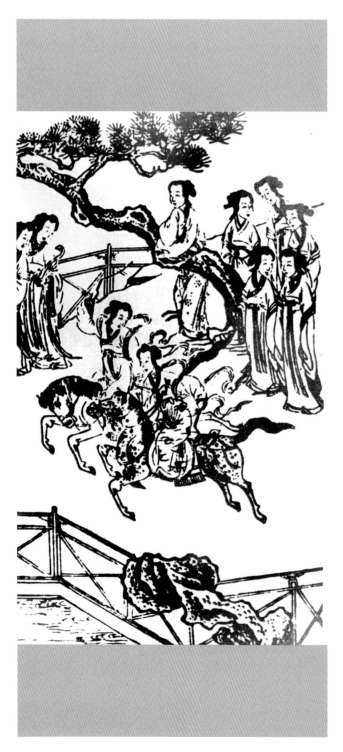

《唐诗艳逸品·仕女赛马图》

明

框：纵 21 厘米，横 126 厘米

《唐诗艳逸品》4 册，明代杨肇祉撰，吴兴闵一栻录评，天启元年（1621）吴兴闵氏刊，朱墨套印本，卷首冠《百美人图》，传为仇英画。此为其中之一幅，描写了仕女赛马的情景。

中国国家图书馆藏

Tang Shi Yan Yi Pin- Shi Nü Sai Ma Tu

Ming Dynasty

Frame: Vertical Length 21 cm/ Horizontal Length 126 cm

Tang Shi Yan Yi Pin (a book on Chinese poetry of Tang Dynasty) is composed of 4 volumes, and was compiled by Yang Zhaozhi in the Ming Dynasty. It was recorded and commented by Min Yishi of Huzhou City, Zhejiang Province (historically called Wuxing) and published in 1621. This picture was printed in red and black. The frontispiece of this book was *Bai Mei Ren Tu* (the picture of a hundred beautiful ladies), which was believed to be painted by Qiu Ying. This picture is part of it, which demonstrates a scene of ladies in horse racing.

Preserved in National Library of China

《宣宗射猎图》

明

纵 29.1 厘米，横 34.6 厘米

该图描绘了明宣宗朱瞻基（1426—1435 年在位）于郊外射猎的情形。

故宫博物院藏

Xuan Zong She Lie Tu

Ming Dynasty

Vertical Length 29.1 cm/ Horizontal Length 34.6 cm

This picture *Xuan Zong She Lie Tu* (Painting of Emperor Hunting) describes a scene of the 5th Ming Emperor, Zhu Zhanji (posthumous title Xuan Zong, reigning 1426 through 1435) hunting in the suburbs.

Preserved in The Palace Museum

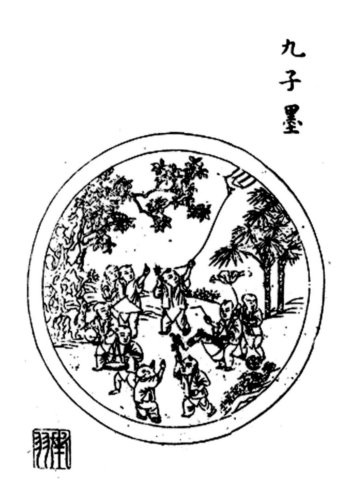

《方氏墨谱·九子墨风筝图》

明

框：宽 13.8 厘米，高 23 厘米

万历十七年（1589）莫荫堂方于鲁刊本。《方氏墨谱》6 卷，明代方于鲁编著，丁云鹏、吴左千、俞仲康画，黄德时刻。这幅《九子墨风筝图》为其中墨谱之一，描写了数名儿童在放风筝、骑竹马游戏的情景。

中国国家图书馆藏

Fang Shi Mo Pu-Jiu Zi Mo Feng Zheng Tu

Ming Dynasty

Frame: Width 13.8 cm/ Height 23 cm

The preserved one was published by Mo Yin Tang Publishing House of Fang Yulu's edition in 1589. *Fang Shi Mo Pu* (a book about ink sticks designs) has 6 chapters and was compiled by Fang Yulu in the Ming Dynasty. It was painted by Ding Yunpeng, Wu Zuoqian and Yu Zhongkang, and carved by Huang Deshi. *Jiu Zi Mo Feng Zheng Tu* is one of the ink stick designs, which depicts some children flying a kite and riding bamboo horses.

Preserved in National Library of China

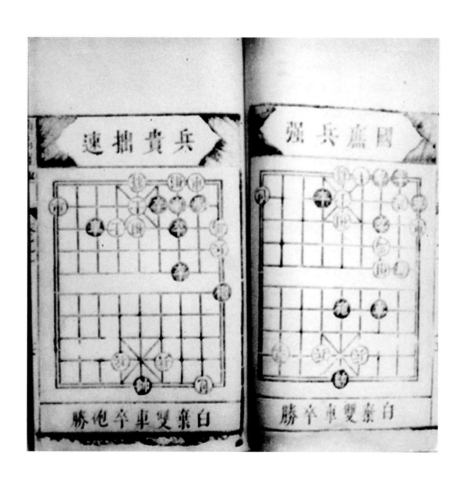

徐芝《适情雅趣》书影

明

竹纸

纵 24.6 厘米，横 14.9 厘米

该书凡 10 卷，10 册，是早期指导象棋实战的重要棋谱之一。保存完整，较为少见。

中国书店藏

Book Photograph of *Shi Qing Ya Qu* by Xu Zhi

Ming Dynasty

Bamboo Paper

Vertical Length 24.6 cm/ Horizontal Length 14.9 cm

This book is composed of 10 chapters in 10 volumes, and is one of the important chess records about the real chess matches in ancient China. It is preserved in complete condition, which makes it rare.

Preserved in China Bookshop

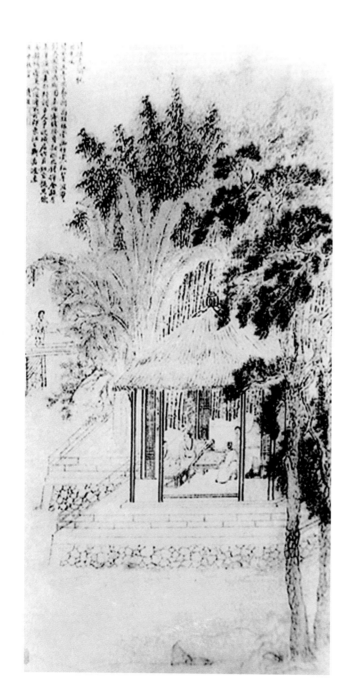

钱古《竹亭对弈图》轴

明

纵 62 厘米，横 32.3 厘米

丛林傍凉亭，二人对坐而弈，颇有清闲情致，旁有二人似在观棋。画上有作者题诗。

辽宁省博物馆藏

Scroll of *Zhu Ting Dui Yi Tu* by Qian Gu

Ming Dynasty

Vertical Length 62 cm/ Horizontal Length 32.3 cm

The painting *Zhu Ting Dui Yi Tu* (Playing Chess at a Bamboo Pavilion) describes in light color that two people are playing chess at a pavilion near the forests, with two other people watching, which looks relaxing and leisurely. There is also a poem on the picture.

Preserved in Liaoning Provincial Museum

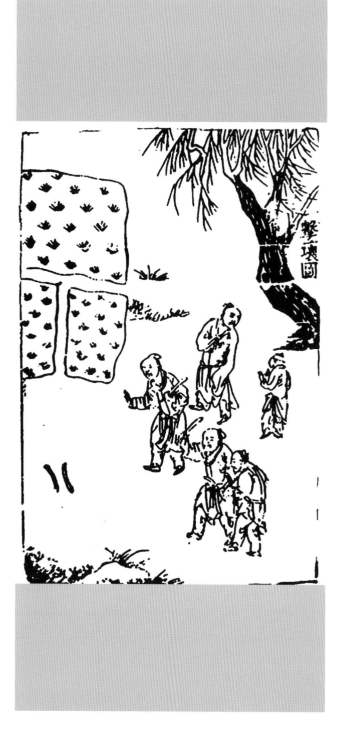

《三才图会·击壤图》

明

万历三十七年（1609）刻本。明代王圻、王思义编著。《击壤图》为其中插图之一。画面中，三人正在大树下各手执一壤（一种前广后锐，长方形，形似履的投掷用具）投击前方地上之壤，其规则是以距离远和投中者为胜。在他们身后，还站有两人，似在观看。

中国国家图书馆藏

San Cai Tu Hui- Ji Rang Tu

Ming Dynasty

The preserved one is the block-printed edition in 1609. *San Cai Tu Hui* (an illustrated ancient Chinese encyclopedia about everything in sky, earth and human world) was compiled by Wang Qi and Wang Siyi in the Ming Dynasty. The painting of *Ji Rang Tu* (a kind of toss game in China) is one of the insets of this book, which describes that three people respectively holding a "Rang" (a quadrate tool with wide front part and sharp end which looks like a shoe) to pitch another "Rang" on the ground. The winner will be the one who hits the goal from the longest distance. There are also two people standing behind them seemingly watching the game.

Preserved in National Library of China

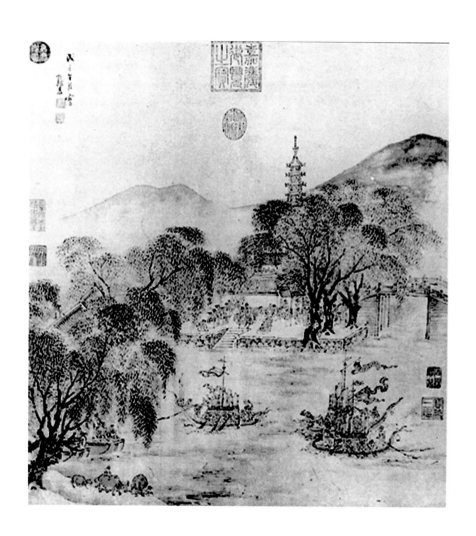

张宏《竞渡图》

明

峭劲秀雅的山峦、树木之间，有两只巨型的龙舟正行驶在广阔的江面上。龙舟上旗帜招展，人们在执桨击水，奋勇竞渡。画面颇具气势，再现了当时龙舟竞渡的盛况。

首都博物馆藏

Jing Du Tu by Zhang Hong

Ming Dynasty

In *Jing Du Tu* (Painting of Boat Racing) there are two huge dragon boats traveling on a wide stretch of river among the graceful mountains and trees. The dragon boats are decked with flags, and people are paddling hard to compete for crossing the river. This magnificent painting demonstrates a visual effect with depth of focus. These dragon-boats and figures are painted freehand and simple, which revives the grand scene of dragon-boat racing.

Preserved in The Capital Museum

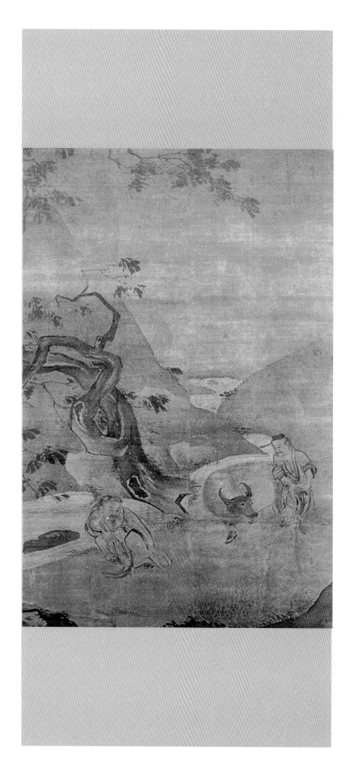

《许由洗耳图》

明

纵 144 厘米，横 101 厘米

明代著名画家吴伟根据许由洗耳的故事而画。

山东省文物总店藏

Xu You Xi Er Tu

Ming Dynasty

Vertical Length 144 cm/ Horizontal Length 101 cm

The famous painter of the Ming Dynasty Wu Wei drew this painting according to the story that Xu You washed his ears to refuse the throne offered by Emperor Yao.

Preserved in Shandong Provincial Store of Cultural Relics

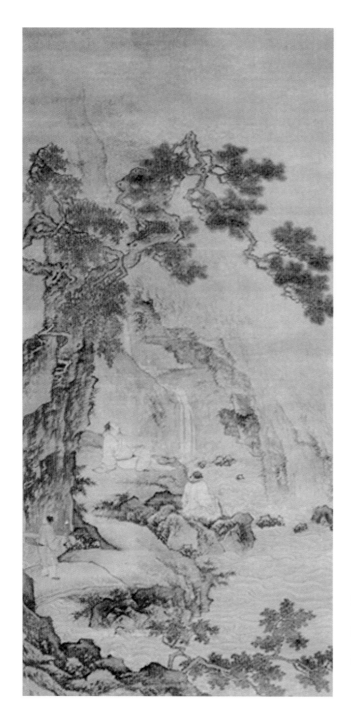

《沧浪濯足图》轴

明

纵 165 厘米，横 82 厘米

绘高士于山间溪流濯足畅怀。画题"周臣"款。

山东博物馆藏

Scroll of *Cang Lang Zhuo Zu Tu*

Ming Dynasty

Vertical Length 165 cm / Horizontal Length 82 cm

This painting *Cang Lang Zhuo Zu Tu* (Foot Washing in Canglang River) describes that Gao Shi is washing his feet and enjoying beautiful scenery in mountain streams. There is an autograph of "Zhou Chen" on the painting.

Preserved in Shandong Museum

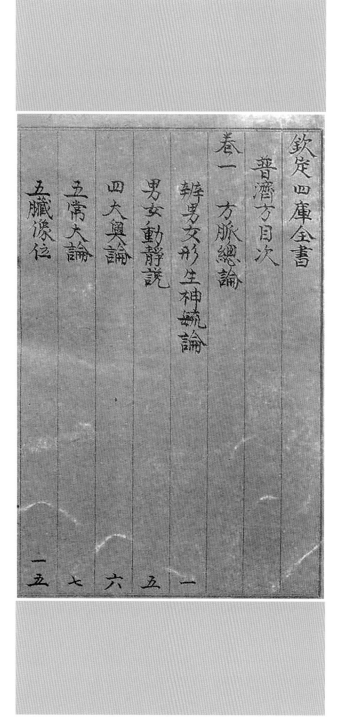

《普济方》书影

明

影抄《四库全书》本。明代朱橚、滕硕、
刘醇等编著。成于永乐四年（1406）。原
书 168 卷，《四库全书》本改订为 426 卷，
1960 论，2175 类，778 法，239 图，61739 方。
《普济方》是我国现存最大的古代方书。

中国中医科学院图书馆藏

Book Photograph of *Pu Ji Fang*

Ming Dynasty

Pu Ji Fang (Prescriptions for Universal Relief), a reference book for medical prescription, was later included in the *Si Ku Quan Shu* (Complete Library in the Four Branches of Literature). *Pu Ji Fang* was written and edited by Zhu Di, Teng Shuo, Liu Chun and so on, and finished in the 4th year of the reign of Emperor Yongle in the Ming Dynasty (1406). The original work had 168 chapters and was later revised into 426 chapters, containing 1,960 analects, 2,175 categories, 778 laws, 239 diagrams and 61,739 medical prescriptions. *Pu Ji Fang* is the most complete one among China's remaining ancient reference books for medical prescriptions.

Preserved in Library of China Academy of Chinese Medical Sciences

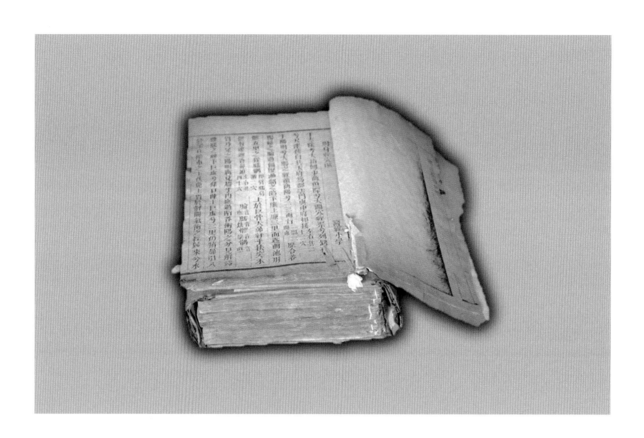

《针灸大成》

明

清乾隆甲寅（1794）文光堂藏版，重刻本。明代杨继洲（济时）撰，清代章廷珪重修。1函10册。保存完整。
陕西中医药大学图书馆调拨。

陕西医史博物馆藏

Zhen Jiu Da Cheng

Ming Dynasty

The book was a reprint edition during the reign of Emperor Qianlong (1974) in the Qing Dynasty, using the engraved blocks stored in Wen Guang Tang. *Zhen Jiu Da Cheng* (Compendium of Acupuncture and Moxibustion) was written by Yang Jizhou (Ji Shi) in the Ming Dynasty and was revised by Zhang Tingui in the Qing Dynasty. It has 10 volumes in 1 case. The collection was allocated from the Library of Shaanxi University of Chinese Medicine and is still well preserved.

Preserved in Shaanxi Museum of Medical History

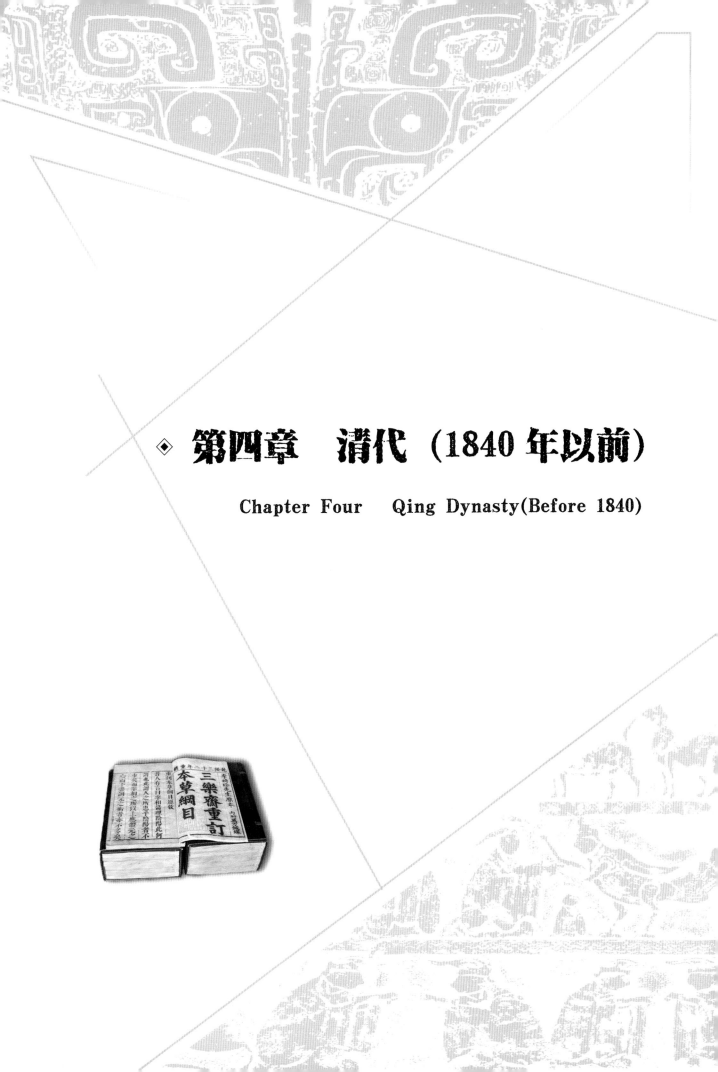

第四章 清代（1840 年以前）

Chapter Four Qing Dynasty(Before 1840)

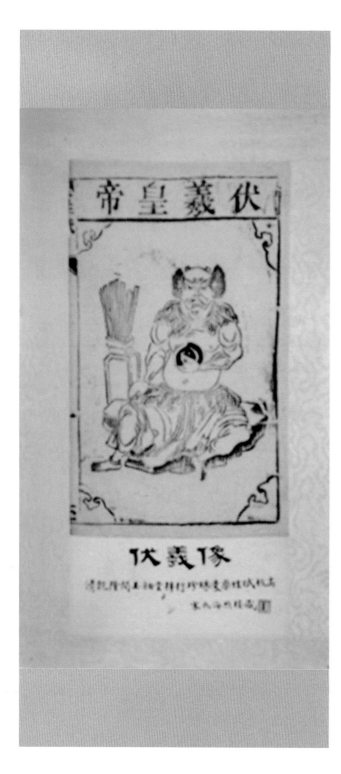

伏羲画像

清

纵 24 厘米，横 11.5 厘米

清乾隆间玉轴堂梓行《珍珠囊药性赋》版画，宋大任仁海煦楼藏。伏羲为旧石器时代中晚期人，中国神话中人类的始祖，相传他作八卦、尝百药、制九针，因此，我国医学界尊奉其为医药学、针灸学的始祖。

广东中医药博物馆藏

Portrait of Fu Xi

Qing Dynasty

Vertical Length 24 cm/ Horizontal Length 11.5 cm

The portrait is a printed painting of *Zhen Zhu Nang Yao Xing Fu* (a medical book on pharmacy) published by Yu Zhou Tang (a Chinese ancient publisher) during the reign of Emperor Qianlong in the Qing Dynasty. Fu Xi was the mythological forefather of human beings living in the middle and late Palaeolithic Age. Legend goes that he created Eight Trigrams, tasted a hundred herbs and made nine kinds of medical needles. Therefore, Chinese medical field considers him to be the founder of Chinese medicine as well as the science of acupuncture and moxibustion.

Preserved in Guangdong Chinese Medicine Museum

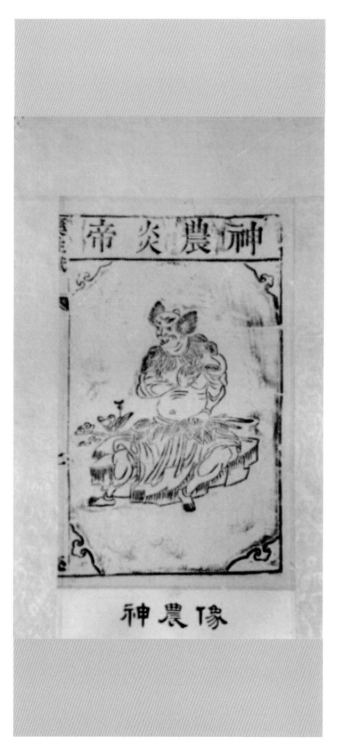

神农炎帝画像

清

纵 24 厘米，横 11.5 厘米

清乾隆间玉轴堂梓行《珍珠囊药性赋》版画，宋大任仁海煦楼藏。神农，一称炎帝，据说为上古三皇五帝之一。《淮南子》载："发明耒耜，散民耕种，并尝百草水泉，令民知所避就，一日而遇七十毒。"所以，传说神农为农业与医药创始人，将医药归于一人，实不可信，然而，反映了先民认识医药的艰辛过程。《神农本草经》乃后世托名。

广东中医药博物馆藏

Portrait of the Yan Emperor Shen Nong

Qing Dynasty

Vertical Length 24 cm/ Horizontal Length 11.5 cm

The portrait is a printed painting of *Zhen Zhu Nang Yao Xing Fu* (a medical book on pharmacy) published by Yu Zhou Tang (a Chinese ancient publisher) during the reign of Emperor Qianlong in the Qing Dynasty. Shen Nong, also called the Yan Emperor, was said to be one of the Three Sovereigns and Five Emperors in ancient mythology. According to *Huai Nan Zi* (a philosophy book in ancient China), "He taught people how to make farming tools and plant crops, and tasted various herbs and spring water to make people know their characters. He used to taste 70 kinds of poisons per day." Therefore, in legend, Shen Nong was the founder of agriculture and medicine with all the achievements under his name, which is unbelievable. However, it reflects the hard process for our ancestors to know the medicine and medication. The book *Shen Nong Ben Cao Jing* (Shen Nong's Herbal Classic) was actually written by descendants in his name.

Preserved in Guangdong Chinese Medicine Museum

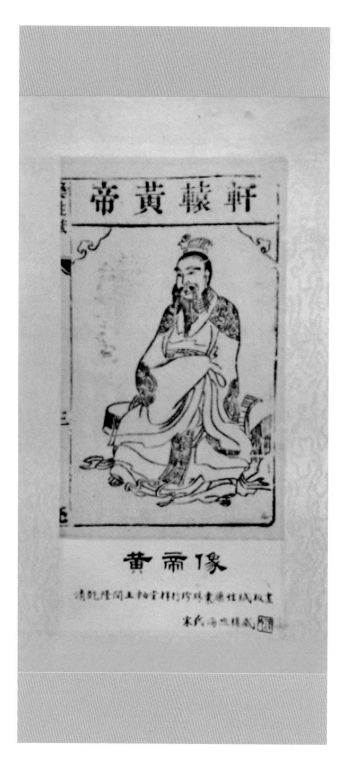

黄帝轩辕画像

清

纵 24 厘米，横 11.5 厘米

清乾隆间玉轴堂梓行《珍珠囊药性赋》版画，宋大任仁海煦楼藏。黄帝，姓公孙（一说姓姬），名轩辕，号有熊氏，传说华夏族的祖先。相传黄帝"使岐伯尝味百草，典医疗疾"，与岐伯、桐君、伯高等讨论医药，刻制九针，始有医药，故后世称中医药为"轩辕之学"或"岐黄之术"。

广东中医药博物馆藏

Portrait of the Yellow Emperor Xuan Yuan

Qing Dynasty

Vertical Length 24 cm/ Horizontal Length 11.5 cm

The portrait is a printed painting of *Zhen Zhu Nang Yao Xing Fu* (a medical book on pharmacy) published by Yu Zhou Tang (a Chinese ancient publisher) during the reign of Emperor Qianlong in the Qing Dynasty. The Yellow Emperor's family name is Gongsun (or Ji in another version), first name, Xuan Yuan and assumed name, Youxiongshi. He was the legendary forefather of the Chinese nationality. Legend goes that "The Yellow Emperor asked Qi Bo to taste various herbs, and then wrote a medical book." He discussed medicine with Qi Bo, Tong Jun and Bo Gao and made nine kinds of medical needles. It is said to be the foundation of traditional Chinese medicine, which, therefore, is also known as "Study of Xuan Yuan" or "Skills of Qi Huang".

Preserved in Guangdong Chinese Medicine Museum

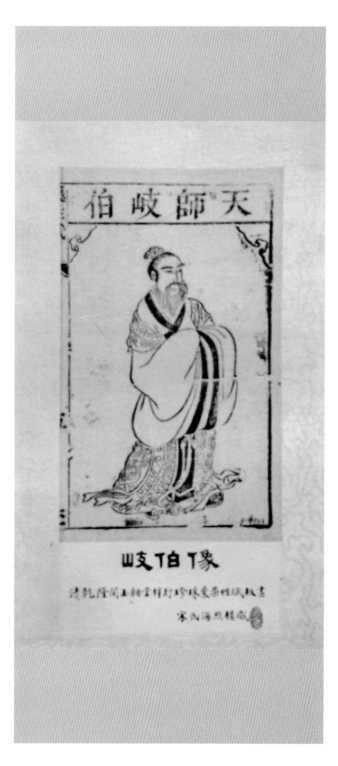

天师岐伯像

清

纵 24 厘米，横 11.5 厘米

清乾隆间玉轴堂梓行《珍珠囊药性赋》版画，
宋大任仁海煦楼藏。《黄帝内经》是由黄帝问、
岐伯答来阐述医理的，因此，后世有以"岐黄"
或"岐黄之术"来称谓中医。

广东中医药博物馆藏

Portrait of a Celestial Master Qi Bo

Qing Dynasty

Vertical Length 24 cm/ Horizontal Length 11.5 cm

The portrait is a printed painting of *Zhen Zhu Nang Yao Xing Fu* (a medical book on pharmacy) published by Yu Zhou Tang (a Chinese ancient publisher) during the reign of Emperor Qianlong in the Qing Dynasty. *Huang Di Nei Jing* (an ancient Chinese medical classic) involved a question-and-answer format between the Yellow Emperor and Qi Bo to state principles of medical science. Therefore, traditional Chinese medicine was also known as "Qi Huang" or "Skills of Qi Huang".

Preserved in Guangdong Chinese Medicine Museum

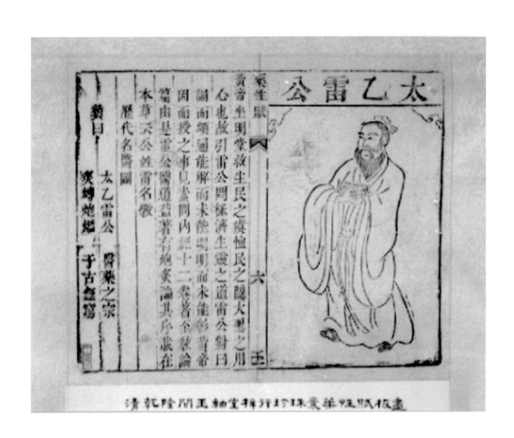

清乾隆间玉轴堂梓行《珍珠囊药性赋》版画

太乙雷公像

清

纵 24 厘米，横 32.5 厘米

清乾隆间玉轴堂梓行《珍珠囊药性赋》版画，宋大任仁海煦楼藏。雷公，南北朝刘宋时人，于药物炮制颇有研究，撰《雷公炮炙论》3 卷，原书已佚，今有辑佚本传世，被后世制药业尊为炮制学鼻祖。

广东中医药博物馆藏

Portrait of Tai Yi Lei Gong

Qing Dynasty

Vertical Length 24 cm/ Horizontal Length 32.5 cm

The portrait is a printed painting of *Zhen Zhu Nang Yao Xing Fu* (a medical book on pharmacy) published by Yu Zhou Tang (a Chinese ancient publisher) during the reign of Emperor Qianlong in the Qing Dynasty. Lei Gong was born in Liu-Song Period of the Northern and Southern Dynasties. Based on his achievement in concocting medicine, he wrote the book *Lei Gong Pao Zhi Lun* (3 chapters). The original book has been lost. Today, a compiled version is still preserved. He was revered as the founder of Chinese medicine processing by descendants of the pharmaceutical industry.

Preserved in Guangdong Chinese Medicine Museum

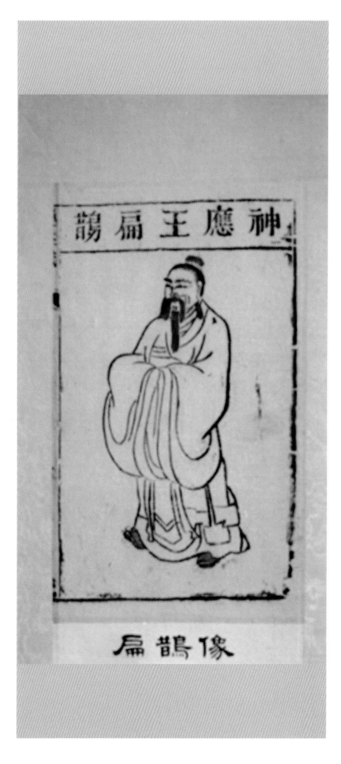

神应王扁鹊像

清

纵 24 厘米，横 11.5 厘米

清乾隆间玉轴堂梓行《珍珠囊药性赋》版画，
宋大任仁海煦楼藏。扁鹊，姓秦，名越人，
战国时渤海郡郑州（今河北）人，通晓医学
各科，尤精诊断，为切脉治病的倡导者。《列
子》记载他曾用"毒药迷人，剖胸探心"，
这是关于麻醉剂的最早记载。

广东中医药博物馆藏

Portrait of the Magic Doctor Bian Que

Qing Dynasty

Vertical Length 24 cm/ Horizontal Length 11.5 cm

The portrait is a printed painting of *Zhen Zhu Nang Yao Xing Fu* (a medical book on pharmacy) published by Yu Zhou Tang (a Chinese ancient publisher) during the reign of Emperor Qianlong in the Qing Dynasty. Bian Que's family name is Qin, and his first name called Yueren. He was born in Bohai Prefecture, Mozhou (in Hebei Province today) in the Warring States Period. Being familiar with all the subjects of medicine, especially on diagnosis, he was the advocator of pulse-taking in treating disease. *Lie Zi* recorded that he ever "anesthetized people with drugs and opened patient's thorax to observe their hearts". This is the earliest record about anesthetics.

Preserved in Guangdong Chinese Medicine Museum

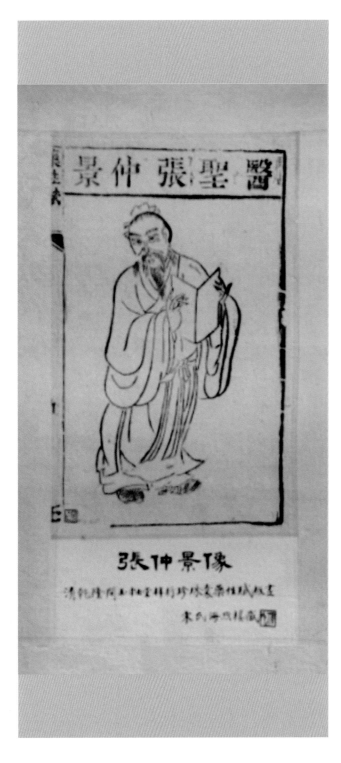

医圣张仲景像

清

纵 24 厘米，横 12 厘米

清乾隆间玉轴堂梓行《珍珠囊药性赋》版画，宋大任仁海煦楼藏。张仲景，东汉南阳人，著《伤寒杂病论》，把汉以前零散的疗法、经验加以整理、发挥，成为中国医学史上药物治疗最有价值的著作，被誉为"方书之祖"。它确定了辨证论治的原则，被后世医家继承、现今注解仲景医作的书籍近千种。

广东中医药博物馆藏

Portrait of Medical Sage Zhang Zhongjing

Qing Dynasty

Vertical Length 24 cm/ Horizontal Length 12 cm

The portrait is a printed painting of *Zhen Zhu Nang Yao Xing Fu* (a medical book on pharmacy) published by Yu Zhou Tang (a Chinese ancient publisher) during the reign of Emperor Qianlong in the Qing Dynasty. Zhang Zhongjing was born in Nanyang County in the Eastern Han Dynasty. His medical monograph, *Shang Han Za Bing Lun* (Treatise on Febrile Disease and Miscellaneous Diseases), is the most valuable work in the history of Chinese medicine, which collected and developed the previously scattered therapies and experience records. It was known as "the foundation of prescriptions", as it established the principle of treating disease in theory of dialectics. And there are almost a thousand other books which interpret and comment his book.

Preserved in Guangdong Chinese Medicine Museum

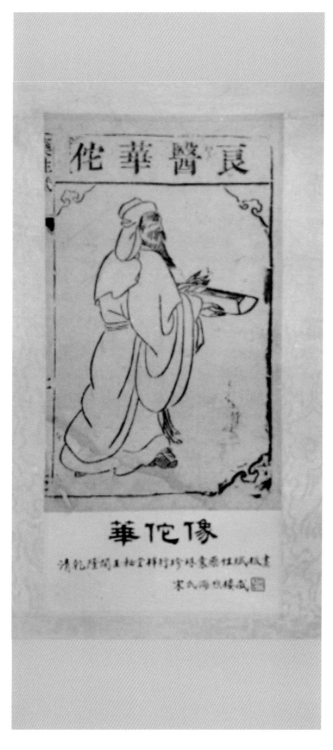

良医华佗像

清

纵 24 厘米，横 11.5 厘米

清乾隆间玉轴堂梓行《珍珠囊药性赋》版画，宋大任仁海煦楼藏。华佗，字元化，东汉沛国谯（今安徽省亳县）人，精医术，尤擅外科，还提倡锻炼身体，自创的"五禽戏"对促进人类健康有积极意义。

广东中医药博物馆藏

Portrait of Hua Tuo

Qing Dynasty

Vertical Length 24 cm/ Horizontal Length 11.5 cm

The portrait is a printed painting of *Zhen Zhu Nang Yao Xing Fu* (a medical book on pharmacy) published by Yu Zhou Tang (a Chinese ancient publisher) during the reign of Emperor Qianlong in the Qing Dynasty. Hua Tuo's courtesy name is Yuanhua, who was born in Qiao County in Kingdom of Pei (now in Boxian County, Anhui Province). He was proficient in medical skills, especially surgery, and was an advocator of physical exercise. "Wu Qin Xi" (Medical Exercises Imitating Movements of Five Animals), which was created by Hua Tuo, is of positive significance to human health.

Preserved in Guangdong Chinese Medicine Museum

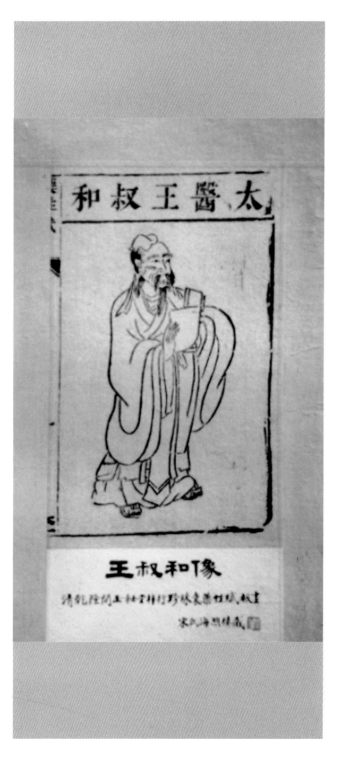

太医王叔和像

清

纵 24 厘米，横 11.5 厘米

清乾隆间玉轴堂梓行《珍珠囊药性赋》版画，宋大任仁海煦楼藏。王叔和，北魏山阳高平（今山东巨野）人，曾任太医令，好经方，并总结魏晋以来脉学成就，著成《脉经》。《脉经》是我国第一部脉学专著。

广东中医药博物馆藏

Portrait of the Imperial Physician Wang Shuhe

Qing Dynasty

Vertical Length 24 cm/ Horizontal Length 11.5 cm

The portrait is a printed painting of *Zhen Zhu Nang Yao Xing Fu* (a medical book on pharmacy) published by Yu Zhou Tang (a Chinese ancient publisher) during the reign of Emperor Qianlong in the Qing Dynasty. Wang Shuhe, born in Gaoping, Shanyang (now in Juye County, Shandong Province), was once an Imperial Physician of the Northern Wei Dynasty with expertise in prescriptions. He compiled the first medical book on sphygmology, *Mai Jing* , by summarizing the relevant achievements from the Wei Dynasty and Jin Dynasty.

Preserved in Guangdong Chinese Medicine Museum

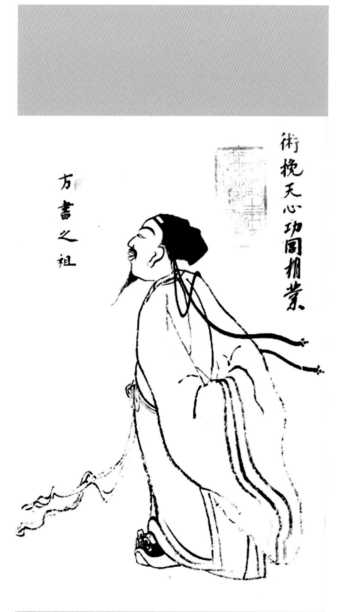

张仲景画像

清

张仲景，名机，东汉末年杰出医学家，南阳郡（今河南南阳）人。医学造诣精深，其学说为中医临证医学奠定了基础；精于临证各科，又倡用灌肠法、坐药、薰法、水渍等治病。后世尊为"医圣"，影响国内外千余年。其《伤寒杂病论》一书，被后世誉为"方书之祖"。

中国医史博物馆藏

Portrait of Zhang Zhongjing

Qing Dynasty

Zhang Zhongjing (another name Zhang Ji) was a talented Chinese physician in the late Eastern Han Dynasty and was born in Nanyang County (now in Nanyang City of Henan Province). He was renowned for the outstanding accomplishments in medical science. His theory laid the foundation for Chinese clinical medicine. As an expert in all sections of clinical medicine, as well as an advocator of the therapies of clyster, suppository, vaporization and water logging, he was regarded as the "sage" of Chinese medicine who had a deep influence on the medical science of China and overseas. The medical book *Shang Han Za Bing Lun* (Treatise on Febrile Disease and Miscellaneous Diseases) was known as the "Foundation of Prescriptions".

Preserved in Chinese Medical History Museum

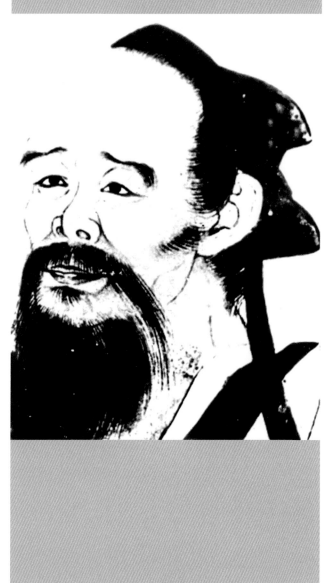

华佗像

清

《历代名贤画像》本。华佗，名旉，字元化，
沛国谯（今安徽省亳县）人，东汉末年杰出
的医学家。精于内、外、妇、针灸等科，其
创用麻沸散进行腹腔手术的事迹尤为著名，
所编之祛病延年的"五禽戏"流传至今。

故宫博物院藏

Portrait of Hua Tuo

Qing Dynasty

This portrait is collected in *Portraits of People of Virtues in the Past Dynasties*. Hua Tuo (styled name Fu and courtesy name Yuanhua) was born in Qiao County in Kingdom of Pei (now in Boxian County, Anhui Province) and was an outstanding physician who lived in the late Eastern Han Dynasty. He was proficient in internal medicine, surgery, gynecology, acupuncture and moxibustion, and he was especially famous for the innovation of using Mafeisan (powder of anesthesia) in celiac operation. His another creation, "Wu Qin Xi" (Medical Exercises Imitating Movements of Five Animals), is still popular now for its function of health maintenance, and is handed down up to now.

Preserved in The Palace Museum

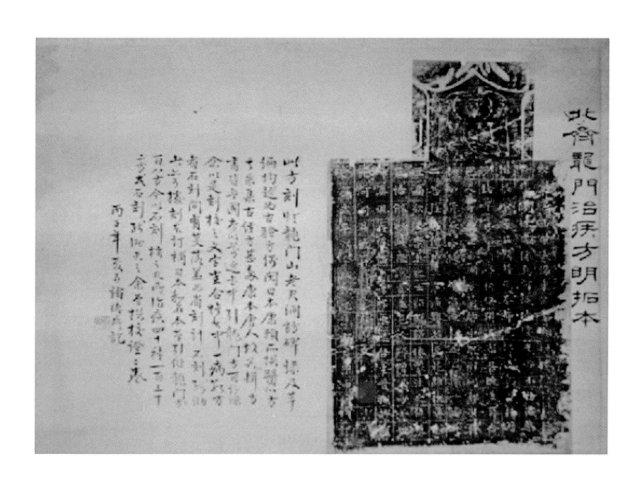

北齐龙门治疾方明拓片（部分）

清初（考证）

此为龙门古药方的明代拓片。洛阳龙门石窟药方是现存最早的古代石刻医方。最早、最详细著录龙门药方是清代王昶 (1725—1807) 的《金石萃编》，王昶将穗藏拓片与《金石萃编》所录药方文字对勘。

广东中医药博物馆藏

Rubbing of the Longmen Prescription in the Northern Qi Dynasty (Partial)

Early Qing Dynasty (verified)

The Ming Dynasty rubbing is an ancient prescription in the Longmen County. The prescriptions found in the Longmen Grottoes in Luoyang City, Henan Province, are the earliest stone-carved ancient prescriptions in existence. The earliest and most detailed book that recorded Longmen prescriptions is *Jin Shi Cui Bian* by Wang Chang (1725–1807) in the Qing Dynasty, which was verified and proofread according to the rubbings preserved in Guangzhou City.

Preserved in Guangdong Chinese Medicine Museum

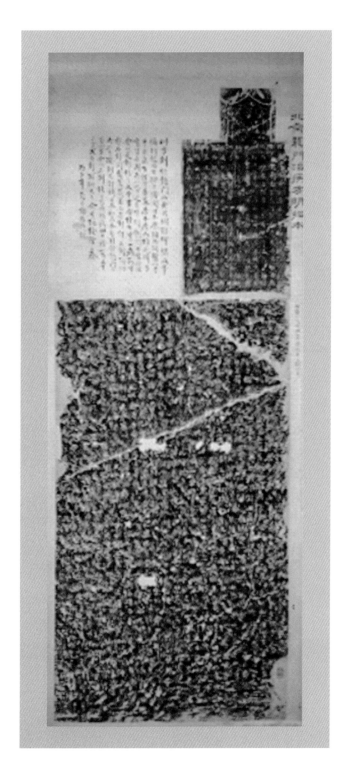

北齐龙门治疾方明拓片

清初（考证）

纵 160 厘米，横 68 厘米

此为龙门古药方的明代拓片。此方刻于洛阳龙门第二十窟（俗称药方洞），属我国最早的石刻药方。河南中医药研究院张金鼎同志致力于中医药研究 40 余年，共补缺字 521 个，复原补全药方 64 首，使龙门石刻药方完整者达 203 首，所治病症 72 种，撰成《龙门石刻药方》一书，是现今龙门方治病最多、所载方剂最全、研究独特的校注本。

广东中医药博物馆藏

Rubbing of the Longmen Prescription in the Northern Qi Dynasty

Early Qing Dynasty (verified)

Vertical Length 160 cm/ Horizontal Length 68 cm

The Ming Dynasty rubbing is an ancient prescription in the Longmen County. This prescription carved in the Longmen Grotto No. 20 (also called the cave of prescriptions), belongs to the earliest stone-carved ones in China. Zhang Jinding, the researcher from Henan Province Chinese Medicine Research Institute, devoted to the study of Chinese medicine for over 40 years. He has repaired 521 damaged characters and completed 64 prescriptions. With his contribution, there have been 203 complete Longmen prescriptions for 72 diseases, which were compiled into *Long Men Shi Ke Yao Fang* (Longmen Stone-carved Prescriptions). The book, with its unique research methods, records the most complete Longmen prescriptions in the largest number.

Preserved in Guangdong Chinese Medicine Museum

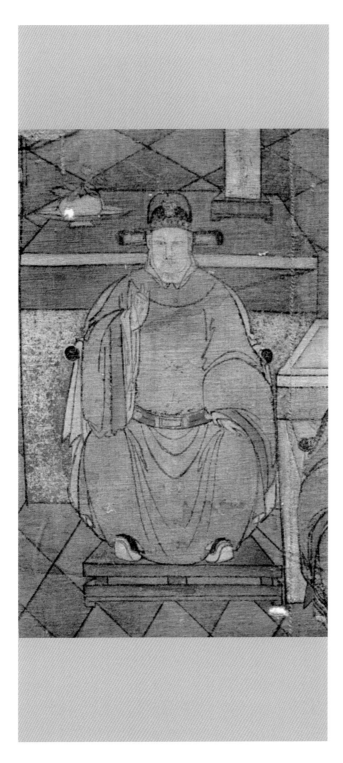

王焘画像

清

王焘（670—755），唐代医药文献学家，撰有《外台秘要》。1975年于王氏故里陕西眉县王家台征集。

陕西医史博物馆藏

Portrait of Wang Tao

Qing Dynasty

Wang Tao (670–755), a famous medical bibliographer in the Tang Dynasty, wrote the medical book of *Wai Tai Mi Yao*. This portrait was collected from Wangjiatai Village, Meixian County, Shaanxi Province, in 1975.

Preserved in Shaanxi Museum of Medical History

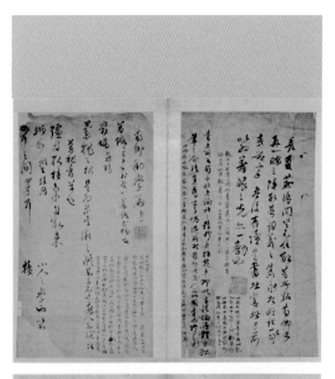

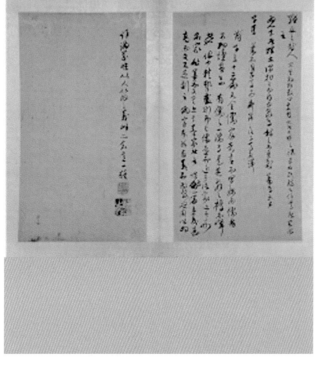

傅山《荀子评注》手稿册

清

纵 46 厘米，横 16 厘米

一册自《劝学篇》起至《王制篇》前半部；
二册自《王制篇》后半部至《天论篇》；三
册自《天论篇》至《正名篇》；四册自《正
名篇》至《性恶篇》。

山西博物院藏

Fu Shan's Manuscript Copies of *Xun Zi Ping Zhu*

Qing Dynasty

Vertical Length 46 cm/ Horizontal Length 16 cm

The first volume starts from *Quan Xue Pian* (Encouraging Learning) to the first half to *Wang Zhi Pian* (On Rules). The second volume starts from the latter part of *Wang Zhi Pian* to *Tian Lun Pian* (On Human and Nature). The third volume starts from *Tian Lun Pian* to *Zheng Ming Pian* (On Naming). And the fourth volume starts from *Zheng Ming Pian* to *E Xing Pian* (On Evil Nature of Human).

Preserved in Shanxi Museum

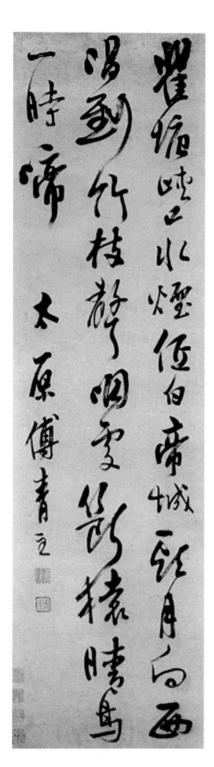

傅青主立轴

清

纵 125.5 厘米，横 35 厘米

此轴书录唐人句，行笔流畅，法度森严，是
其早期代表作之一。

上海中医药博物馆藏

Calligraphy Scroll by Fu Qingzhu

Qing Dynasty

Vertical Length 125.5 cm/ Horizontal Length 35 cm

This calligraphy work records a poem in the Tang Dynasty, which is of smooth strokes and a solemn artistic effect. It was one of Fu's early masterpieces.

Preserved in Shanghai Museum of Traditional Chinese Medicine

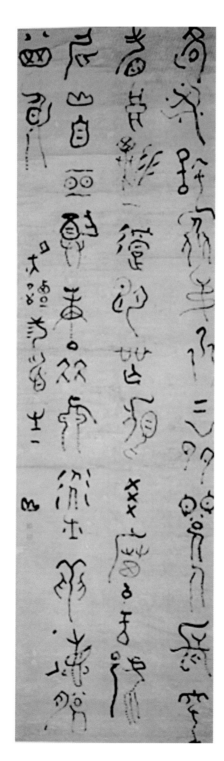

傅山草篆夜读三首之一诗轴

清

纵 330 厘米，横 97 厘米

草篆写五律一首"何必许家第，乃云多阅人，
长空看高翼，一过即无痕。世庙私王号，尼
山自圣尊，唐虞真道士，龙德脱其身。夜读
三首之一，山"。钤"傅山印""青主"两印。
此诗收录于傅山文集《霜红龛集》中。

山西博物院藏

Poem Scroll of Fu Shan's Cursive and Seal Script

Qing Dynasty

Vertical Length 330 cm/ Horizontal Length 97 cm

This calligraphy work is a poem of five-character octave in cursive and seal script, which was one of the three poems Fu Shan was reading at night. There are two signets of "Fu Shan" and "Qing Zhu" on it. This poem was recorded in Fu Shan's work collection *Shuang Hong Kan Ji*.

Preserved in Shanxi Museum

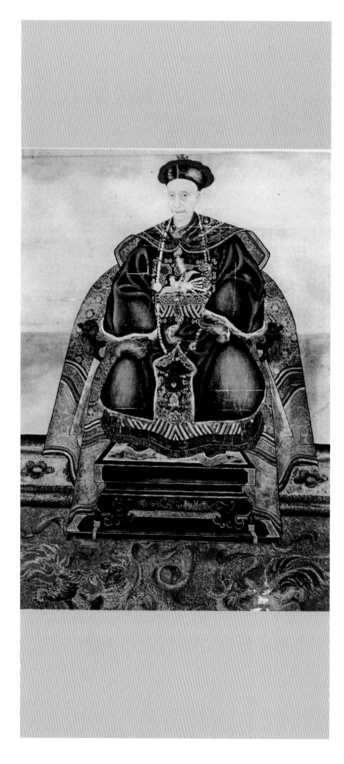

陈尧道画像

清

长 90 厘米，宽 66 厘米

陈尧道，字素中，陕西三原永清里人，清初
医家。著有《伤寒辨证》《痘疹辨证》等书。
陕西三原征得。

陕西医史博物馆藏

Portrait of Chen Yaodao

Qing Dynasty

Length 90 cm/ Width 66 cm

Chen Yaodao, with the courtesy name of Suzhong, was born in Yongqingli Village, Sanyuan County in Shaanxi Province. As a well-known doctor in the early Qing Dynasty, he was the author of *Shang Han Bian Zheng* (a book on the differentiation of febrile diseases) and *Dou Zhen Bian Zheng* (a book on the differentiation of rash and pox). This portrait was collected in Sanyuan County, Shaanxi Province.

Preserved in Shaanxi Museum of Medical History

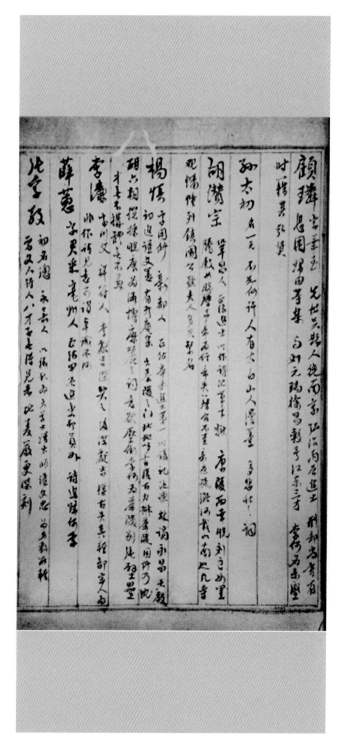

徐大椿手迹

清

徐大椿（1693—1771），名大业，字灵胎，晚号洄溪老人，江苏吴江人，清代医家。工文辞，精医学。著有《难经经释》《医学源流论》等书。图为其手书历代文人事迹的真迹。

中国医史博物馆藏

Handwriting of Xu Dachun

Qing Dynasty

Xu Dachun (1693–1771), with a courtesy name of Lingtai, given name of Daye and a pseudonym of Huixi Laoren in old age, was a physician in the Qing Dynasty. He was born in Wujiang City in Jiangsu Province and was good at writing and skillful in medicine. He wrote the medical books of *Nan Jing Jing Shi* (an interpretation work for the book *Cannon on Eighty-One Difficulty Issues*) and *Yi Xue Yuan Liu Lun* (a medical book with comments and personal opinions on medicine). This picture is his authentic handwriting, which introduces stories of different scholars in history.

Preserved in Chinese Medical History Museum

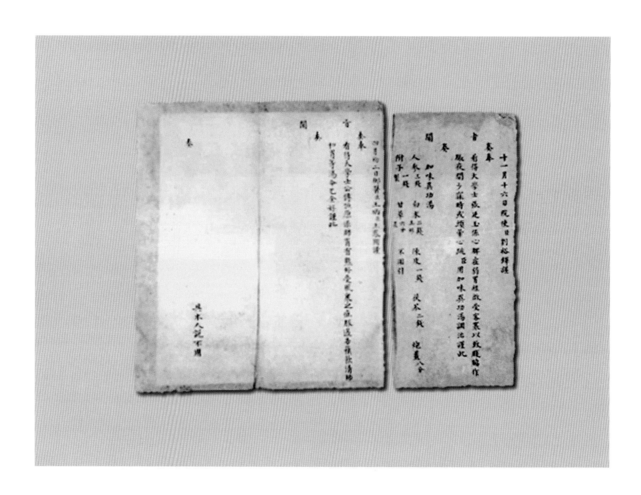

刘裕铎诊病脉案笺

清

图右件系御医刘裕铎为大学士张廷玉诊病的脉案笺。张廷玉（1672—1755），字衡臣，安徽桐城人。康熙、雍正、乾隆三朝大臣，前后居官 50 年，曾任纂修《明史》总裁官。

故宫博物院藏

Liu Yuduo's Diagnosis Note Paper

Qing Dynasty

The collection on the right is the diagnosis note paper for the great intellectual Zhang Tingyu written by the Imperial Physician Liu Yuduo. Zhang Tingyu (1672–1755), with the courtesy name of Hengchen, was born in Tongcheng City, Anhui Province. He had been an official for fifty years through the reigns of Emperor Kangxi, Emperor Yongzheng and Emperor Qianlong in the Qing Dynasty, and also presided the compiling project of *Ming Shi* (History of the Ming Dynasty).

Preserved in The Palace Museum

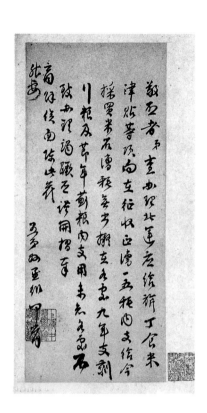

孙星衍尺牍

清

左图：纵 18 厘米，横 33 厘米

右图：纵 23 厘米，横 8.5 厘米

孙星衍（1753—1818），字渊如，阳湖（今江苏武进）人。清代著名学者。精于经史文字之学，旁及诸子百家及岐黄之术，尤精校勘。曾辑《神农本草经》。

上海中医药博物馆藏

Letters of Sun Xingyan

Qing Dynasty

Left: Vertical Length 18 cm/ Horizontal Length 33cm

Right: Vertical Length 23 cm/ Horizontal Length 8.5 cm

Sun Xingyan (1753–1818), with the courtesy name of Yuanru, was born in Yanghu County (now Wujin County, Jiangsu Province). He was a famous scholar of the Qing Dynasty who had a good mastery of traditional classics from different schools, as well as traditional Chinese medicine. He was especially skillful at emendation and edited the medical book *Shen Nong Ben Cao Jing* (Shen Nong's Herbal Classic).

Preserved in Shanghai Museum of Traditional Chinese Medicine

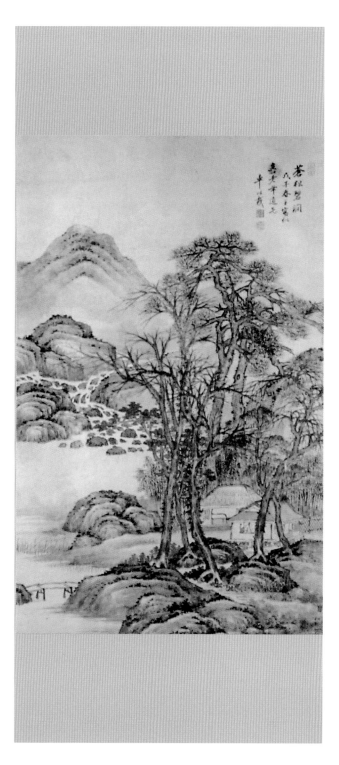

车以载山水画

清

画芯：长 96.8 厘米，宽 61.8 厘米

车以载于清道光（1828）年所绘，画面为水墨苍松碧涧。车以载，明末清初医家，详情待考。已裱成卷轴，纸张泛黄，画面有污迹。1958 年入藏。

中华医学会/上海中医药大学医史博物馆藏

A Landscape Painting by Che Yizai

Qing Dynasty

Painting: Length 96.8 cm/ Width 61.8 cm

This painting with calligraphy, painted by Che Yizai in 1828, depicts green pines and clear mountain stream. Che Yizai was a doctor in the late Ming and early Qing Dynasties. Detailed information of him is not clear now. The painting had been mounted as a scroll. There can be seen yellow discoloration and smudges on the paper. It was collected in 1958.

Preserved in Chinese Medical Association/ Museum of Chinese Medicine, Shanghai University of Traditional Chinese Medicine

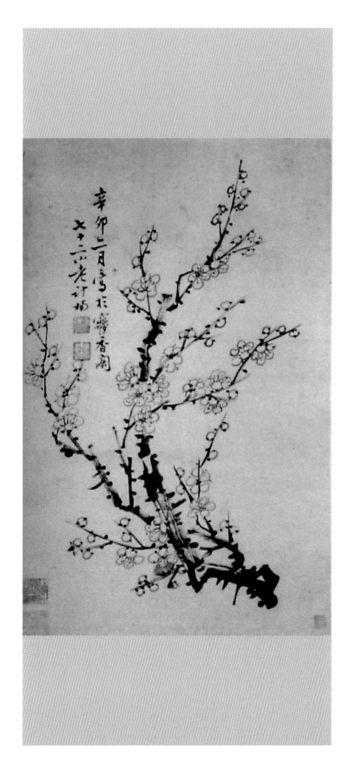

计寿乔墨梅真迹图

清

画芯：长 48 厘米，宽 30.2 厘米

计寿乔于清道光十一年（1831，辛卯年）二月，在梦香阁绘墨梅图，钤"计楠"之印。计寿乔，名计楠，字寿乔，秀水（今嘉兴）人，清代医家。博雅工诗，自学成医，精谙医理，擅长妇科，著有《客尘医话》3 卷。已裱成卷轴，纸张泛黄，画面有污迹。1958 年入藏。

中华医学会 / 上海中医药大学医史博物馆藏

Ji Shouqiao's Authentic Work of Ink Plum Blossom

Qing Dynasty

Painting: Length 48 cm/ Width 30.2 cm

The ink plum blossom painting was painted by Ji Shouqiao in 1831 in Mengxiang Pavilion. The seal of "Ji Nan" was affixed to it. Ji Shouqiao (given name Jinan and courtesy name Shouqiao) was born in Xiushui (now Jiaxing County), who was an erudite doctor and poet in the Qing Dynasty. Being his own teacher, Ji finally became an expert at medicine, especially gynecology. He had written *Ke Chen Yi Hua* (a 3-chapter medical book about the author's opinion and clinical experience of the medicine). The painting had been mounted as a scroll. There can be seen yellow discoloration and smudges on the paper. It was collected in 1958.

Preserved in Chinese Medical Association/ Museum of Chinese Medicine, Shanghai University of Traditional Chinese Medicine

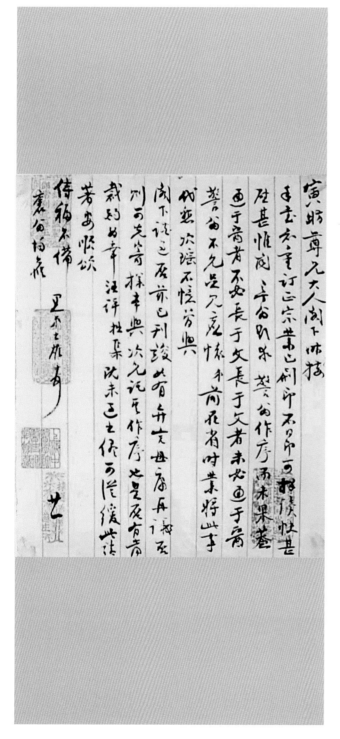

王孟英笔札

清

纵 23 厘米，横 18.9 厘米

该藏由红格白纸黑墨书成，是王孟英为出版
医书而给"寅昉"的信函。文末有王孟英的
别号"士雄"落款。并钤"云锦耀记监制邓
常利号苏庄""邓耀乡号货真价实"印章等。
王孟英（1808—1868），名士雄，浙江海宁人，
清代著名医家。精研医理，擅医温热病，著
作多收入《潜斋医学丛书》。保存基本完好，
纸张泛黄。1961 年入藏。

中华医学会 / 上海中医药大学医史博物馆藏

Writing of Wang Mengying

Qing Dynasty

Vertical Length 23 cm/ Horizontal Length 18.9 cm

This writing material is a letter written with black ink on a piece of rectangle white paper with red grids, affixed with some seals about the author. This letter was written by Wang Mengying to Yin Fang for the publication of a medical book. Wang Mengying (1808–1868) (given name Shixiong) was born in Haining County, Zhejiang Province. He was a famous doctor in the Qing Dynasty, who mastered medical knowledge and was proficient in treating the epidemic febrile disease. Most of his works were collected in *Qianzhai Medical Series* (Qianzhai was the name of Wang Mengying's study). The letter is mostly well preserved with some yellow discoloration. It was collected in 1961.

Preserved in Chinese Medical Association/ Museum of Chinese Medicine, Shanghai University of Traditional Chinese Medicine

王孟英笔札

清

纵 23 厘米，横 18.9 厘米

该藏由红格白纸黑墨书成，是王孟英为出版医书而给"寅昉"的信函。文末有王孟英的别号"士雄"落款。保存基本完好，纸张泛黄。1961 年入藏。

中华医学会 / 上海中医药大学医史博物馆藏

Writing of Wang Mengying

Qing Dynasty

Vertical Length 23 cm/ Horizontal Length 18.9 cm

This writing material is a letter written with black ink on a piece of rectangle white paper with red grids, affixed with the seal about the author. This letter was written by Wang Mengying to Yin Fang for the publication of a medical book. The letter is mostly well preserved with some yellow discoloration. It was collected in 1961.

Preserved in Chinese Medical Association/ Museum of Chinese Medicine, Shanghai University of Traditional Chinese Medicine

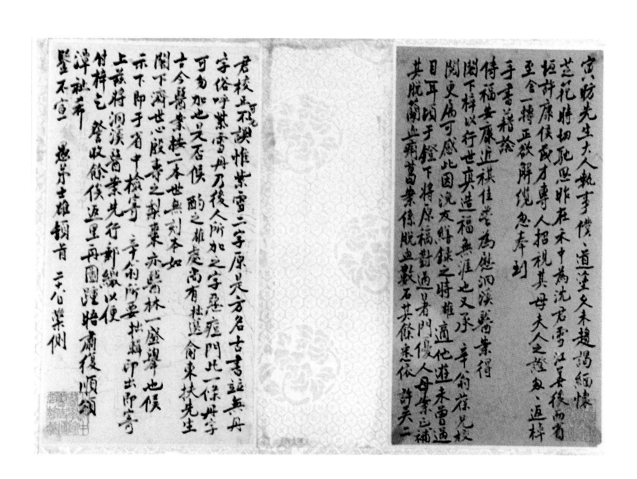

王士雄尺牍

清

纵 16.3 厘米，横 26 厘米

王士雄，字孟英，号梦隐，清代医家。尤擅温病，著有《温热经纬》《霍乱论》等书。

上海中医药博物馆藏

A Letter of Wang Shixiong

Qing Dynasty

Vertical Length 16.3 cm/ Horizontal Length 26 cm

Wang Shixiong (courtesy name Mengying, and style name Mengyin) was a doctor in the Qing Dynasty. He was skilled in treating the epidemic febrile disease and had written books such as *Wen Re Jing Wei* (Compendium on Epidemic Febrile Diseases) and *Huo Luan Lun* (Treatise on Cholera).

Preserved in Shanghai Museum of Traditional Chinese Medicine

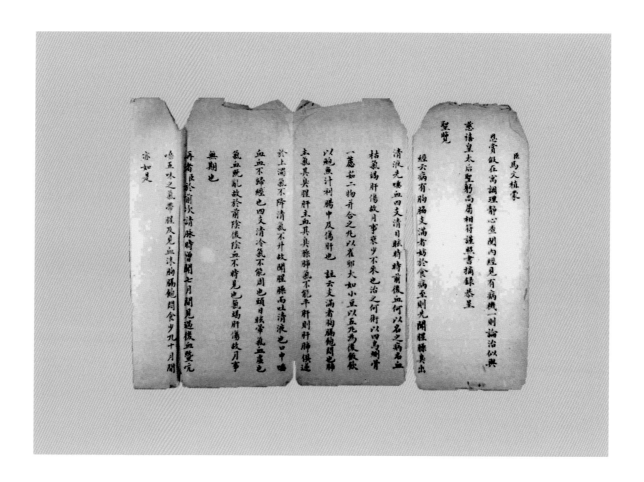

马培之诊治慈禧奏折

清

马文植(1820—1903)，字培之，江苏武进人。近代名中医。出身六世医家，精于内、外等科证治，尤擅外科。光绪六年(1880)由江苏巡抚吴元炳荐为慈禧治病。此为其结合《黄帝内经》理论探索慈禧病患治疗方案的奏折。

故宫博物院藏

Ma Peizhi's Treatment Memorial for Cixi

Qing Dynasty

Ma Wenzhi (1820–1903), courtesy name Peizhi, born in Wujin, Jiangsu Province, was a famous doctor in the modern times. From a family of six generations of doctors, Ma was an expert in internal medicine and surgery, especially in surgery. In 1880, he was recommended by Wu Yuanbing, the provincial governor of Jiangsu Province, as the doctor for Empress Dowager Cixi. The memorial was the therapeutic regimen for Cixi's disease based on the theory of *Huang Di Nei Jing* (Internal Canon of the Yellow Emperor).

Preserved in The Palace Museum

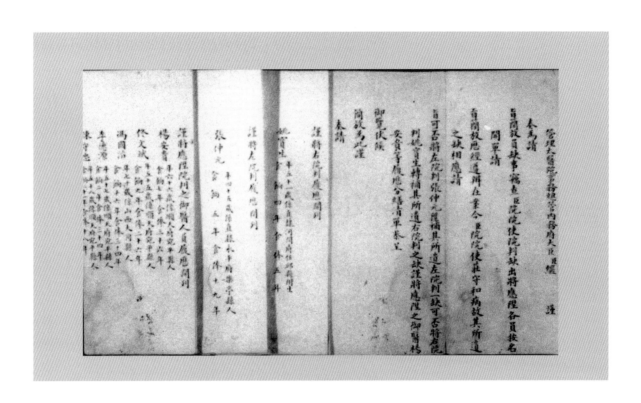

太医院为升补院判事奏折

清

光绪朝太医院院史庄守和病故，太医院奏请原左院判张仲元升补院使，而由原右院判升补其缺，另请升补原御医杨安贵等数人为院判，此为所拟升补人员之履历清单。

故宫博物院藏

Memorial of Imperial Hospital

Qing Dynasty

In the years of the reign of Emperor Guangxu, Yuanshi (administrator of the Imperial Academy of Medicine) Zhuang Shouhe succumbed to an illness. The Imperial Hospital presented this memorial for the promotion of Zhang Zhongyuan and Yang An'gui, etc. This memorial was a resumed list of the promoted personnel.

Preserved in The Palace Museum

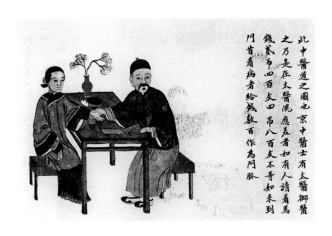

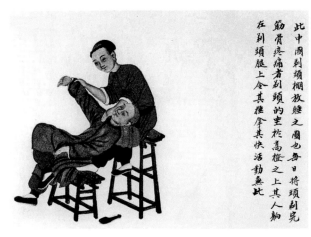

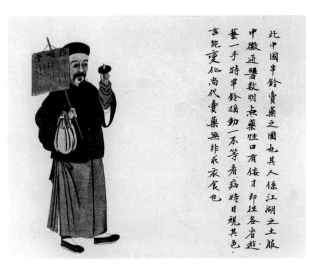

《北京民间生活彩图》书影

清

民间艺人的绘画稿本。画工精细，包罗面广，反映了当时的社会风貌。此选录有关医药卫生的三幅图：图1为《医道图》，描绘了医者治病的场景；图2为《剃头放睡图》，描绘了剃头师傅为顾客按摩的情形；图3为《串铃卖药图》，描绘了民间医生走街串巷卖药治病的形象。

中国医史博物馆藏

Book Photograph of *Color Drawings of Folk Life in Beijing*

Qing Dynasty

This book was the painting manuscript of folk artisans. The exquisite paintings reflect various living styles and social features of that time. The excerption contains three pictures about medicine and health: Picture 1 *Art of Healing* depicts the scene of a doctor treating a patient. Picture 2 *Barber's Massage* depicts the situation in which a qualified shaver is massaging a customer. Picture 3 *Selling Drugs with a Ring-shaped Bell* depicts the image of a folk doctor selling drugs while wandering from street to street.

Preserved in Chinese Medical History Museum

何绍基书药王庙碑拓片

清

河北涿州于明嘉靖中曾建有药王庙，后于清道光中重修。图为清代官吏、学者、书法家何绍基（1799—1873）在药王庙重修竣工后于道光二十五年（1845）所书的庙碑之拓片。

中国医史博物馆藏

Calligraphy Rubbing of Yaowang Temple Stele by He Shaoji

Qing Dynasty

Yaowang (God of Medicine) Temple was established in Zhuozhou County, Hebei Province, during the reign of Emperor Jiajing of the Ming Dynasty and was renovated during the reign of Emperor Daoguang of the Qing Dynasty. This is the rubbing of temple stele calligraphy of He Shaoji (1799–1873), who was a government official, scholar and calligrapher in the Qing Dynasty. The calligraphy was written in 1845, when the renovation of the temple was completed.

Preserved in Chinese Medical History Museum

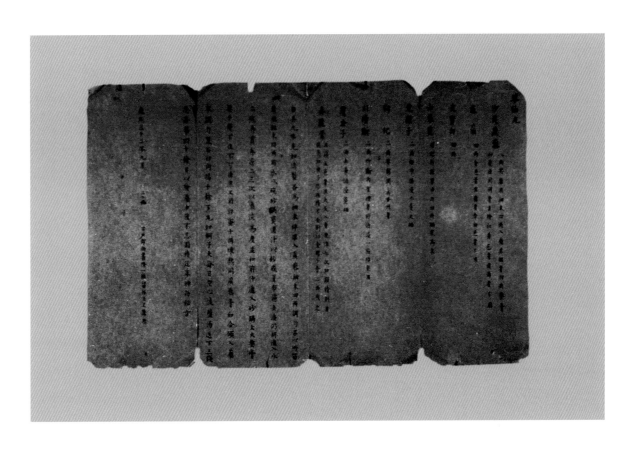

康熙朝官吏呈奏验方折

清

康熙朝户部尚书王鹰于康熙三十二年九月二十九日呈奏的"萃仙丸"方。

故宫博物院藏

Memorial of Imperial Official to Emperor Kangxi

Qing Dynasty

This memorial of the recipe of "Cui Xian Wan" (a pill for the treatment of kidney deficiency) was presented by Wang Ying, the Minister of the Ministry of Revenue, on September 29 of the 32nd year of the reign of Emperor Kangxi of the Qing Dynasty.

Preserved in The Palace Museum

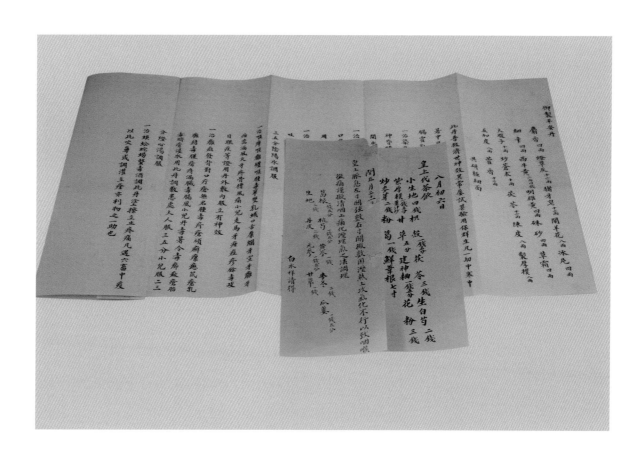

御生堂药方

清

宽 12 厘米，高 24 厘米

此为御生堂白永祥御医给皇帝开具的御方。

北京御生堂中医药博物馆藏

Prescriptions of Yu Sheng Tang

Qing Dynasty

Width 12 cm/ Height 24 cm

It was the prescriptions of the Emperor given by the Imperial Physician Bai Yongxiang of Yu Sheng Tang.

Preserved in Chinese Medicine Museum of Beijing Yu Sheng Tang Drugstore

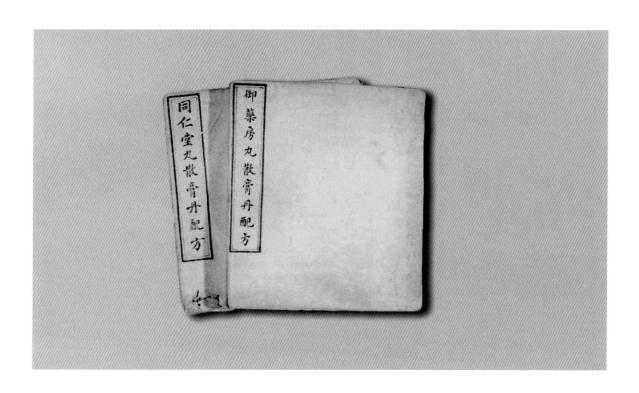

雍正朝御药房及同仁堂丸散膏丹配方

清

同仁堂为清代御前当差药店，故其配方本在宫中亦存档。

故宫博物院藏

Recipes from the Imperial Drug Institution and Tong Ren Tang

Qing Dynasty

Tong Ren Tang was the imperial drugstore in the Qing Dynasty, so its files of recipes were collected in the palace as well.

Preserved in The Palace Museum

道光朝乾清宫药房药材贮销清单

清

清宫各药房均常贮各种药材以备医疗之用，此为上述药材库贮销使用清单。

故宫博物院藏

Crude Drugs Lists of Pharmacy in Palace of Heavenly Purity of Emperor Daoguamg

Qing Dynasty

Pharmacies in all palaces of the Qing Dynasty used to store various kinds of crude drugs for treatment of diseases. These lists recorded the storage and use of those crude drugs.

Preserved in The Palace Museum

鳖 甲 處處有 牡 蠣 出江浙 真 珠 出廣東

石決明 出廣東 青 蒿 出荊州 骨碎補 出江南

秫 米 處處有 苾 米 出真定 大 棗 出青州

木 瓜 出宣州 檀 香 出雲南 淡 菜 出東南海中

十大功勞 出江南 沉 香 出交趾 枳 殼 出河南

枳 實 出河南江北 九香蟲 出貴州 黄 柏 出漢中

清宫应用各地进贡药材档

清

清宫供医用之中药材均由各地进贡，宫中对此要求甚为严格，各药之出处均有记载。此件为该档中部分地道药材之出处记录。

故宫博物院藏

The File of Tribute Crude Drugs in Qing Palaces

Qing Dynasty

Traditional Chinese crude drugs for medical purposes in palaces of the Qing Dynasty were tributes from various regions, so the drugs were strictly controlled. Provenances of all the crude drugs were recorded. This collection was a record of the provenances of some authentic crude drugs in the file.

Preserved in The Palace Museum

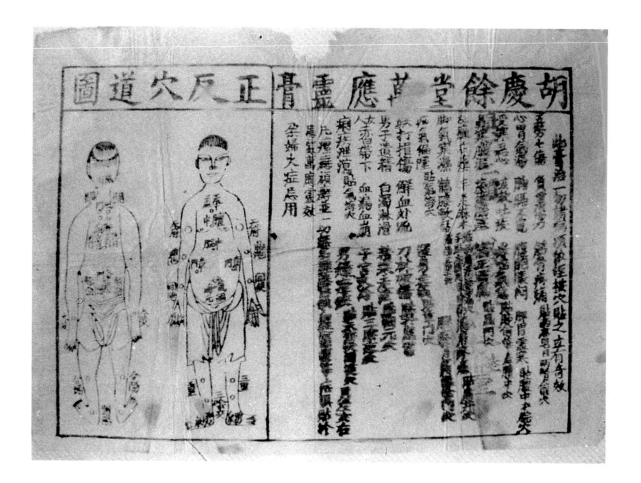

"胡庆余堂"仿单

清

其为杭州著名药店"胡庆余堂"的"万应灵膏"的广告说明书。

史常永供稿

A Drug Instruction from "Hu Qing Yu Tang"

Qing Dynasty

It was an advertised instruction of Wanyingling Ointment made by Hu Qing Yu Tang, a famous drugstore in Hangzhou City.

Provided by Shi Changyong

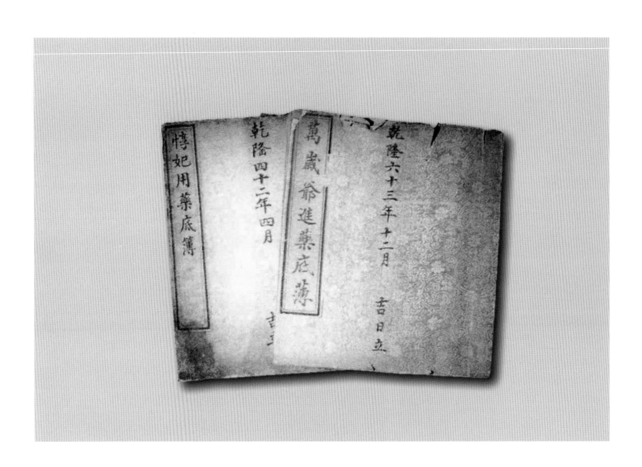

乾隆及惇妃脉案档

清

乾隆六十三年十二月《万岁爷进药底簿》及乾隆四十二年四月《惇妃用药底簿》之封面。乾隆在位60年，后3年为太上皇，乾隆六十三年即嘉庆三年 (1798)。

故宫博物院藏

Medical Records of Emperor Qianlong and Consort Dun

Qing Dynasty

These are covers of *Wan Sui Ye Jin Yao Di Bu* (File of Drug Administration for the Emperor) in lunar December of the 63rd year of the reign of Emperor Qianlong of the Qing Dynasty and *Dun Fei Yong Yao Di Bu* (File of Drug Administration for Consort Dun) in lunar April of the 42nd year of the reign of Emperor Qianlong. Emperor Qianlong was on the throne for sixty years and retired for the following three years, so the 63rd year of the reign of Emperor Qianlong was the third year of the reign of Emperor Jiaqing (1798).

Preserved in The Palace Museum

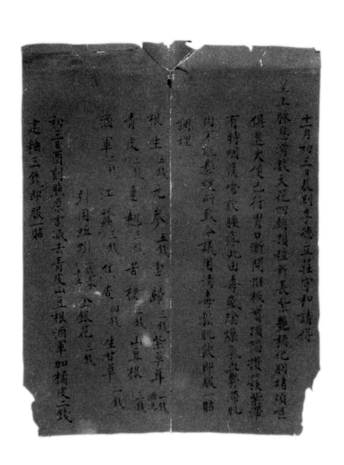

同治帝天花脉案档

清

相传同治帝罹患梅毒，而据同治十三年十月至十一月《万岁爷天花喜进药用药簿》记录，可知实患天花并发感染。此为同治帝患天花时的脉案档一则。

故宫博物院藏

Medical Records of Smallpox of Emperor Tongzhi

Qing Dynasty

It was said that Emperor Tongzhi had suffered from syphilis, while according to the record of during October and November in the 13th year of the reign of Emperor Tongzhi, it could be proved that Emperor Tongzhi was actually affected by smallpox combined with infections. This is one of the medical records of this disease of Emperor Tongzhi.

Preserved in The Palace Museum

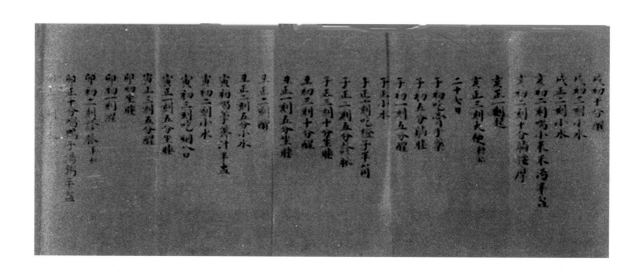

恭亲王护病记录

清

中医护理是一门科学性较强、很细致的学问。此件恭亲王护病记录可资说明。记录中对患者的服药、进食水果与饮料、排便、吸烟、诊脉、入睡的时间及饮食养生，均有详细记录，以供医患两者参照。

故宫博物院藏

A Nursing Record of Prince Kung

Qing Dynasty

Traditional Chinese medical nursing is a scientific and meticulous subject, which can be proved by a nursing record of Prince Kung. This nursing record kept detailed information of the patient's drug administration, intake of fruits and beverages, defecation, smoking, pulses, time to fall asleep and dietary regimen, which provided references both for the doctor and the patient.

Preserved in The Palace Museum

法国驻京医官多德福为光绪会诊脉案档

清

光绪帝素体羸弱，常有病患。戊戌政变后一个月，病情加剧，传法国医官多德福入宫会诊。此为光绪二十四年九月四日脉案档，处方中应用了地黄末等。

故宫博物院藏

Medical Record of Emperor Guangxu Written by French Doctor

Qing Dynasty

Emperor Guangxu's health was in feeble condition and he often had sickness. One month after the Wu-xu Coup, Emperor Guangxu's disease aggravated. The French doctor in Beijing, Duo Defu (the Chinese name of the French doctor), had a group consultation for him. The picture was the medical record written by Duo Defu on the date of 4th of September in the 24th year of the reign of Emperor Guangxu. The medical record also includes the prescription of using the powder of radices rehmanniae as well as other medicines.

Preserved in The Palace Museum

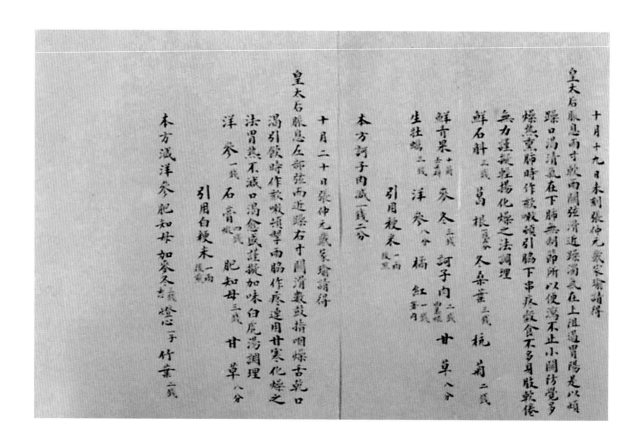

慈禧用西洋参脉案档

清

清宫脉案中，多见应用西洋参者。在慈禧脉案中亦然，如御医张仲元、戴家瑜等诊治慈禧疾患之处方中均有。

故宫博物院藏

Medical Record of Cixi Having American Ginseng

Qing Dynasty

In the medical records that were stored in the Qing palaces, many people had the history of having American Ginseng. Empress Dowager Cixi's medical file also recorded the history of using American Ginseng. Imperial Physicians like Zhang Zhongyuan and Dai Jiayu, had ever prescribed American Ginseng for Empress Dowager Cixi.

Preserved in The Palace Museum

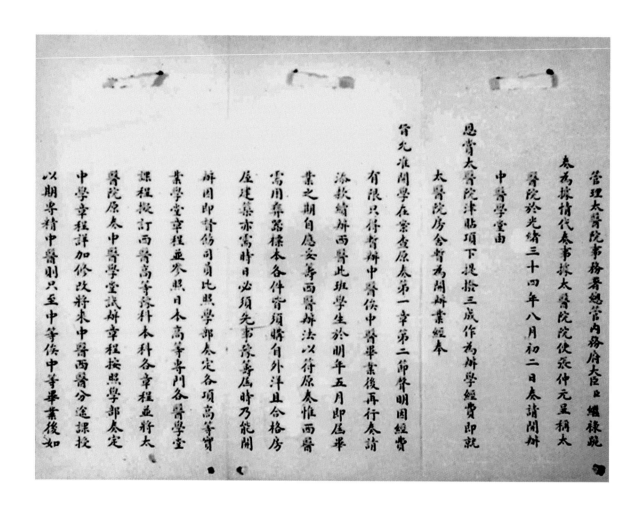

光绪朝太医院关于中医学堂增设西医课之奏折

清

光绪朝太医院院使张仲元与御医李崇光就中医学堂是否增设西医课程一事有不同看法，遂分别奏请光绪帝裁夺。此为奏折中之一件。

故宫博物院藏

Memorial to Emperor Guangxu about Course of Western Medicine

Qing Dynasty

Envoy of Imperial Hospital Zhang Zhongyuan and Imperial Physician Li Chongguang had different opinions on whether to offer the course of Western Medicine in the Chinese Medicine School. They respectively submitted their own memorials to Emperor Guangxu for his arbitration. The picture was one of the two memorials.

Preserved in The Palace Museum

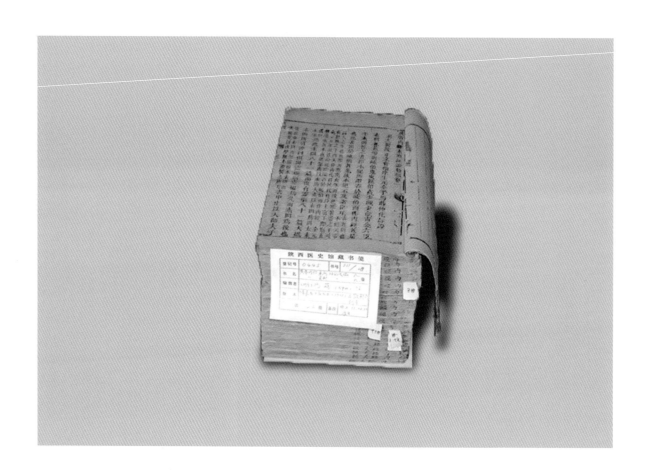

《黄帝内经灵枢注证发微》九卷，附《素问遗篇》

清

古歙鲍漱芳〔席芬〕慎余堂刻本。明代马莳〔仲化〕注，24册。保存完整。陕西中医药大学图书馆调拨。

陕西医史博物馆藏

Huang Di Nei Jing Ling Shu Zhu Zheng Fa Wei

Qing Dynasty

The book was a block-printed edition by Bao Shufang's Shen Yu Tang (the name of an ancestral hall). The annotations of the book were added by Ma Shi in the Ming Dynasty. Containing 24 volumes, the books were allocated from the Library of Shaanxi University of Chinese Medicine and is still well preserved.

Preserved in Shaanxi Museum of Medical History

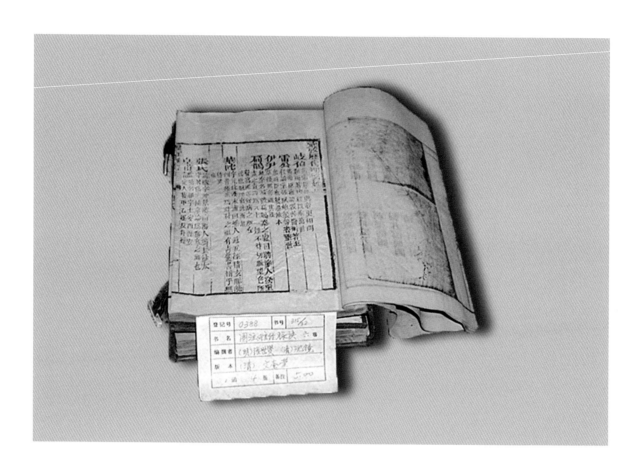

《图注难经脉诀》

清

文奎堂刻本。明代张世贤图注，清代沈镜删注，1函4册。保存完整。陕西中医药大学图书馆调拨。

陕西医史博物馆藏

Tu Zhu Nan Jing Mai Jue

Qing Dynasty

Tu Zhu Nan Jing Mai Jue (an illustrated medical book) shown in the picture was a block-printed edition of Wen Kui Tang (the name of a book store). The drawing statement was added by Zhang Shixian in the Ming Dynasty and was revised by Shen Jing in the Qing Dynasty. The book had 4 volumes in 1 case. The books were allocated from the Library of Shaanxi University of Chinese Medicine and is still well preserved.

Preserved in Shaanxi Museum of Medical History

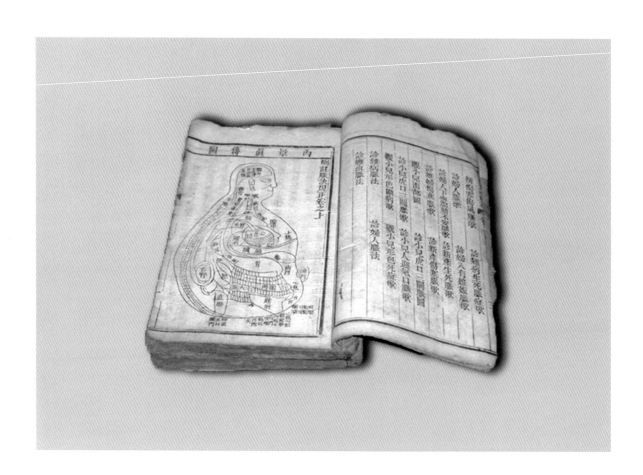

《图注难经脉诀》

清

起凤堂刻本。明代张世贤图注，清代沈镜删注。2 册。书皮有"张维翰"三字。保存完整。陕西中医药大学图书馆调拨。

陕西医史博物馆藏

Tu Zhu Nan Jing Mai Jue

Qing Dynasty

Tu Zhu Nan Jing Mai Jue (an illustrated medical book) shown in the picture was a block-printed edition of Qi Feng Tang. The drawing statement was added by Zhang Shixian in the Ming Dynasty and was revised by Shen Jing in the Qing Dynasty. The book has 2 volumes. There are three Chinese characters "Zhang Wei Han" on the book cover. The books were allocated from the Library of Shaanxi University of Chinese Medicine and is still well preserved.

Preserved in Shaanxi Museum of Medical History

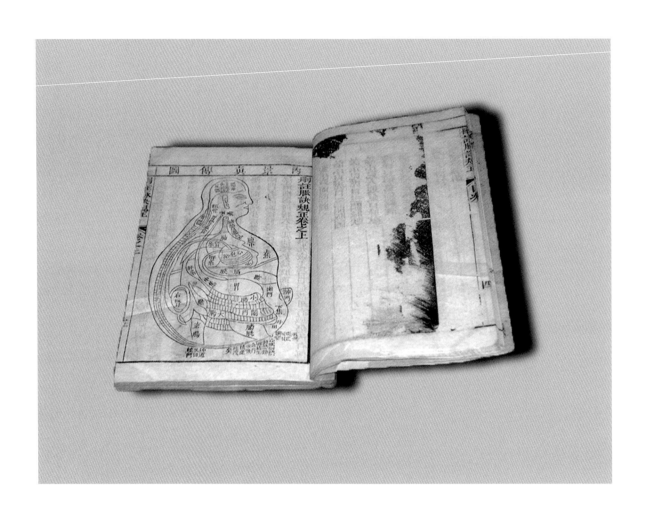

《图注难经脉诀》

清

小酉山房刻本。明代张世贤图注，清代沈镜删注。1 册。保存完整。陕西中医药大学图书馆调拨。

陕西医史博物馆藏

Tu Zhu Nan Jing Mai Jue

Qing Dynasty

Tu Zhu Nan Jing Mai Jue (an illustrated medical book) shown in the picture was a block-printed edition of Xiao You Shan Fang. The drawing statement was added by Zhang Shixian in the Ming Dynasty and was revised by Shen Jing in the Qing Dynasty. The book has only 1 volume. The book was allocated from the Library of Shaanxi University of Chinese Medicine and is still well preserved.

Preserved in Shaanxi Museum of Medical History

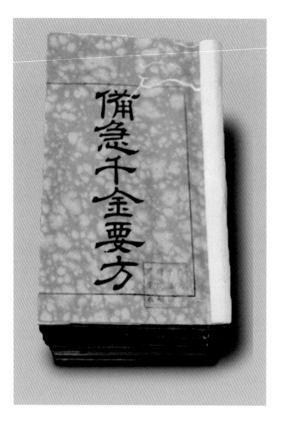
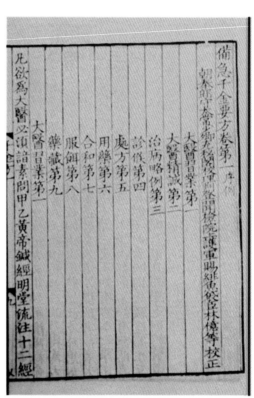

《备急千金要方》一套十二册

清

长 30 厘米，宽 18.5 厘米，重 2455 克

清光绪江户医学影北宋本（光绪戊寅夏五购自东瀛），唐代著名医学家孙思邈所著，30 卷，详细阐述了医学理论、医方，与《备急千金方》合称《千金方》，代表了盛唐医学先进水平，在我国影响极大，并在亚洲广为传播。日本医学界誉《千金方》为"人类之至宝"。

广东中医药博物馆藏

Bei Ji Qian Jin Yao Fang (1 Set/ 12 Volumes)

Qing Dynasty

Length 30 cm/ Width 18.5 cm/ Weight 2,455 g

The books were the copy print of those in the Northern Song Dynasty and purchased from Japan in 1878 during the reign of Emperor Guangxu. *Bei Ji Qian Jin Yao Fang* (Thousand-gold Prescriptions for Emergency)was written by Sun Simiao, a famous doctor in the Tang Dynasty, and it has 30 chapters with detailed explanations of medical theory and prescriptions, which represented the advanced medical level in the Tang Dynasty and had a great impact in China as well as the whole Asian area. It was praised by Japanese doctors as the "most valuable treasure of human being".

Preserved in Guangdong Chinese Medicine Museum

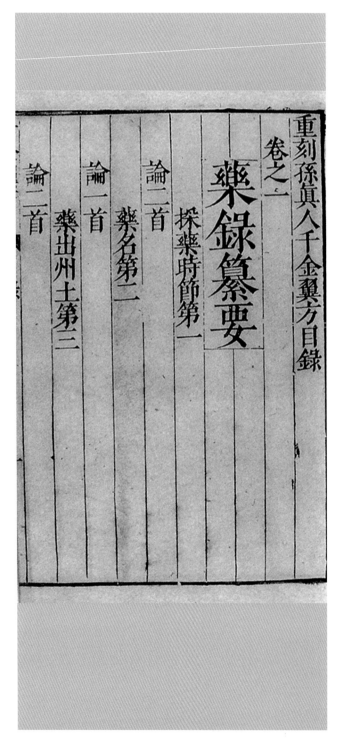

《千金翼方》书影

清

清刻本。孙思邈著。30 卷。为《千金要方》
的续编，故称"翼方"。书中辑录药物 800 余种，
有些是唐以前未收录的新药和外来药物。书中
对内、外各种病症的诊治在《千金要方》基
础上均有增补，并收载了当时医家所秘藏的
《伤寒论》内容，选录了《千金要方》所未
载的古代方剂 2000 余首。

中国中医科学院图书馆藏

Book Photograph of *Qian Jin Yi Fang*

Qing Dynasty

The book was a block-printed edition in the Qing Dynasty. It was written by Sun Simiao, a famous doctor in the Tang Dynasty, and contains 30 chapters. It is called "Yi Fang" (prescriptions of wings) as it is the supplement of *Qian Jin Yao Fang* (Invaluable Prescriptions for Ready Reference). There are more than 800 kinds of medicines recorded in this book, some of which were not recorded until the Tang Dynasty and some were introduced from abroad. On the basis of *Qian Jin Yao Fang*, the book supplemented the treatment of various diseases. It also recorded the secret collection of *Shang Han Lun* (Treatise on Febrile Diseases) and more than 2,000 ancient prescriptions which were not included in *Qian Jin Yao Fang.*

Preserved in Library of China Academy of Chinese Medical Sciences

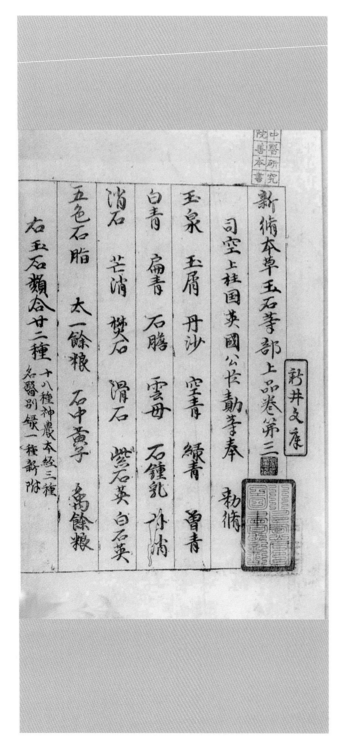

《新修本草》书影

清

光绪己丑年（1899）德清傅氏影刻唐卷子本。

本书系唐代苏敬等 20 余人奉旨于显庆二年

至显庆四年（657—659）编成。共 54 卷。

成书后由政府颁行全国，并流传日本、朝鲜

等国。现存唐人手写之敦煌卷子本及日本古

卷子抄本。

中国中医科学院图书馆藏

Book Photograph of *Xin Xiu Ben Cao*

Qing Dynasty

The book *Xin Xiu Ben Cao* (New Edition of Materia Medica) was the copy-print edition of Fu's in 1899. The original book was compiled by over 20 people in the Tang Dynasty including Su Jing under the order of the Emperor Xianqing during 657–659. Containing 54 chapters, it was spread nationwide and even to Japan and the Korean Peninsula. Now the preserved editions are the Dunhuang edition written by people in the Tang Dynasty and the ancient hand-written copies in Japan.

Preserved in Library of China Academy of Chinese Medical Sciences

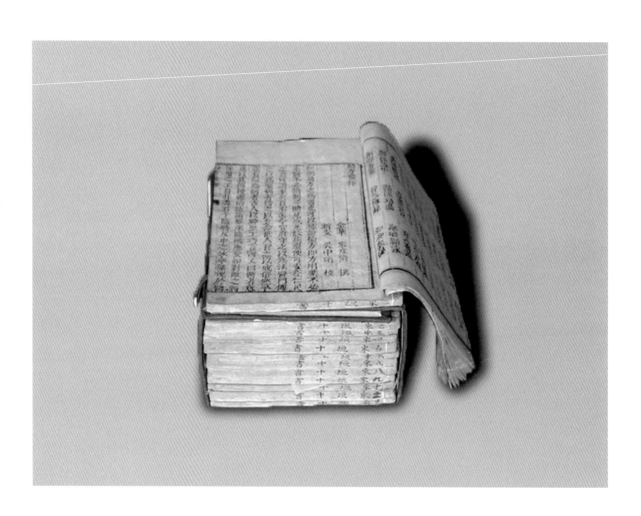

《东垣十书》

清

金元诸家撰，明代王肯堂（宇泰）订正。1 函 12 册。敦化堂藏版，子目共收 12 种医书。保存完整。陕西中医药大学图书馆调拨。

陕西医史博物馆藏

Dong Yuan Shi Shu

Qing Dynasty

The book was compiled by many scholars in the Jin and Yuan Dynasties and revised by Wang Kentang in the Ming Dynasty. The book has 12 volumes in 1 case and contains 12 medical books in the sub-category. It was a precious collection of Dun Hua Tang. The books were allocated from the Library of Shaanxi University of Chinese Medicine and is still well preserved.

Preserved in Shaanxi Museum of Medical History

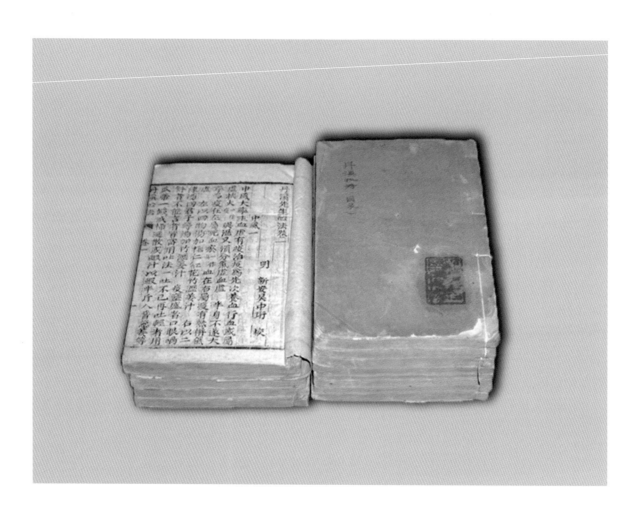

《丹溪心法》附余六种

清

文奎堂刻本。12 册。附余子目中有金代李杲、明代戴元礼所撰之医书。陕西中医药大学图书馆调拨。

陕西医史博物馆藏

Dan Xi Xin Fa and Six Appendixes

Qing Dynasty

The book *Dan Xi Xin Fa* (Danxi's Mastery of Medicine) was a block-printed edition of Wen Kui Tang. The book has 12 volumes. The six appendixes include medical books written by Li Gao in the Jin Dynasty and Dai Yuanli in the Ming Dynasty. The books were allocated from the Library of Shaanxi University of Chinese Medicine.

Preserved in Shaanxi Museum of Medical History

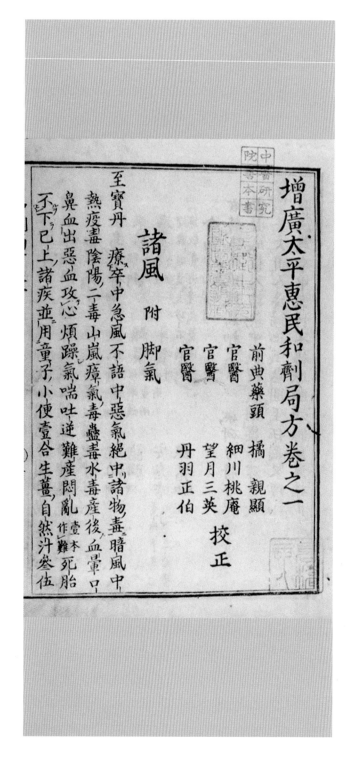

《太平惠民和剂局方》书影

清

日本享保十五年（1730）橘亲显等校刻本。

本书系北宋政府所设药局拟定的制剂规范，

原名《和剂局方》。后经医官陈承、裴宗元、

陈师文等校正，分 5 卷 21 门，279 方。南

宋时书名随药局名更换而改称《太平惠民和

剂局方》，并陆续增订为 10 卷 14 门，共收

788 方。

中国中医科学院图书馆藏

Book Photograph of *Tai Ping Hui Min He Ji Ju Fang*

Qing Dynasty

Tai Ping Hui Ming He Ji Ju Fang (Prescriptions of Peaceful Benevolent Dispensary) was a block-printed edition by Ju Qinxian in 1730. The book was the pharmaceutics standard set up by the drug administration of the Northern Song government, with the original name, *He Ji Ju Fang*. Then revised by doctors Chen Cheng, Pei Zhongyuan, Chen Shiwen and so on, the book recorded 279 prescriptions in 21 subjects and 5 chapters. In the Southern Song Dynasty, its name was changed to the present one due to the name change of the drug administration. It finally recorded 788 prescriptions in 14 subjects and 10 chapters.

Preserved in Library of China Academy of Chinese Medical Sciences

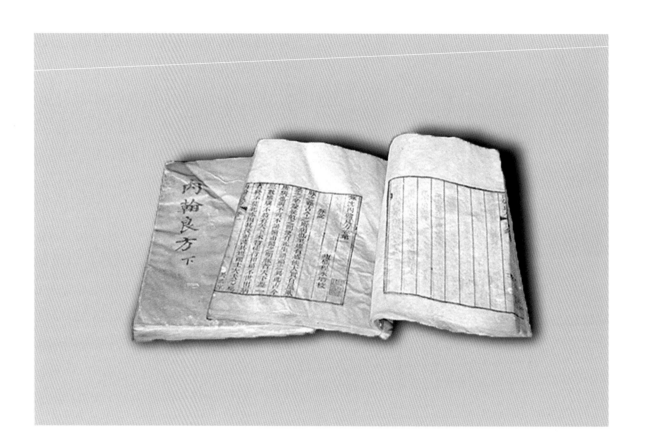

《苏沈内翰良方》十卷

清

清乾隆五十九年甲寅（1794）修敬堂刻六醴斋医书本。宋代苏轼、沈括撰。2册。保存完整。陕西中医药大学图书馆调拨。

陕西医史博物馆藏

Su Shen Nei Han Liang Fang (10 Chapters)

Qing Dynasty

Containing 2 volumes, the book is a block-printed edition published by Xiu Jing Tang and Liu Li Zhai in 1794. *Su Shen Nei Han Liang Fang* (Effective Prescriptions by Su and Shen) was written by Su Shi and Sheng Kuo in the Song Dynasty. The books were allocated from the Library of Shaanxi University of Chinese Medicine and is still well preserved.

Preserved in Shaanxi Museum of Medical History

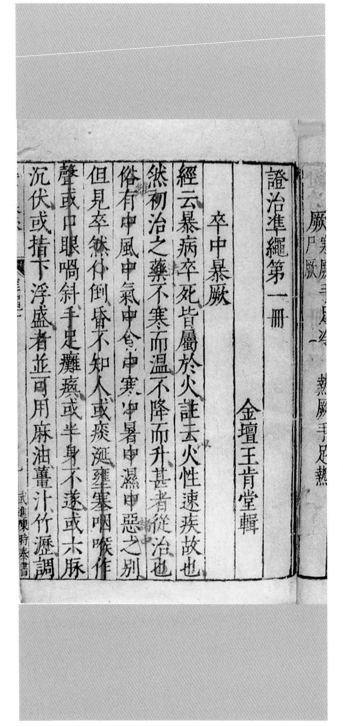

《证治准绳》书影

清

康熙三十八年己卯（1699）金坛虞氏补修本。

王肯堂编撰。又名《六科准绳》，44卷，

分为《杂病证治准绳》等6种。

中国中医科学院图书馆藏

Book Photograph of *Zheng Zhi Zhun Sheng*

Qing Dynasty

This edition was revised by Yu from Jintan County in year 1699. *Zheng Zhi Zhun Sheng*, another name *Liu Ke Zhun Sheng* (Standards of Diagnosis and Treatment), was compiled by Wang Kentang. It has 44 chapters in six categories.

Preserved in Library of China Academy of Chinese Medical Sciences

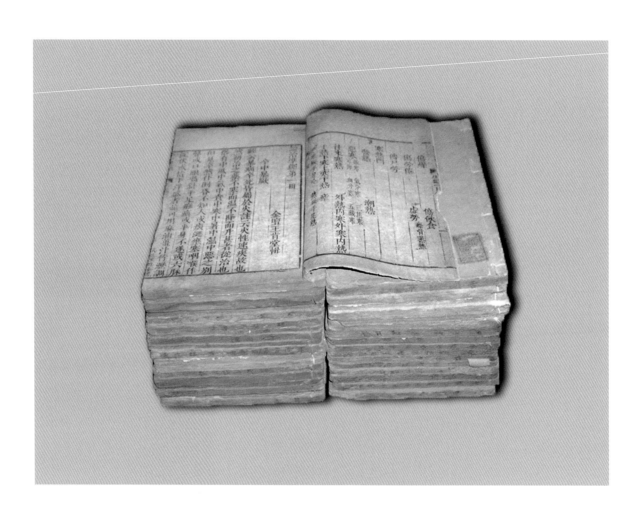

《六科证治准绳》

清

清康熙三十八年（1699）金坛虞氏修补刻本，武进陈时泰书。明代王肯堂撰。34 册。有残缺。陕西中医药大学图书馆调拨。

陕西医史博物馆藏

Liu Ke Zheng Zhi Zhun Sheng

Qing Dynasty

Containing 34 volumes, this edition was revised by Yu from Jintan County, hand-written by Chen Shitai from Wujin County and printed in 1699. The book *Liu Ke Zheng Zhi Zhun Sheng* (Principles in Diagnosing and Treating Six Categories of Diseases) was originally compiled by Wang Kentang in the Ming Dynasty. The books were allocated from the Library of Shaanxi University of Chinese Medicine and is incomplete.

Preserved in Shaanxi Museum of Medical History

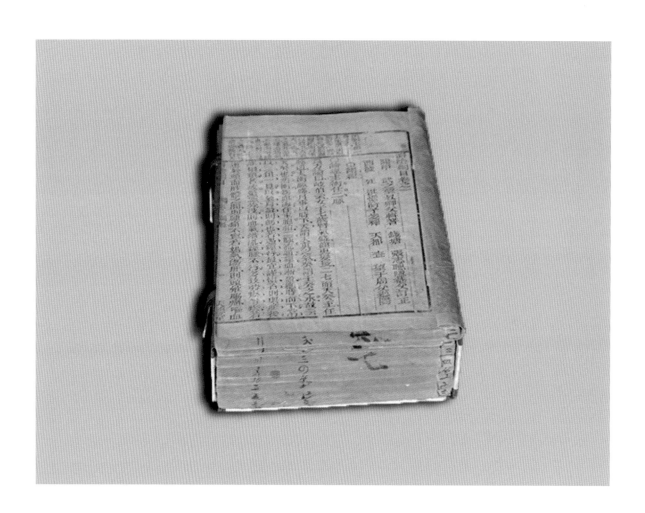

《济阴纲目》十四卷，附：保生碎事

清

清天德堂刻本。明代武之望，清代汪琪（憺漪子，右之）笺释。1 函 8 册。保存完整。陕西中医药大学图书馆调拨。

陕西医史博物馆藏

Ji Yin Gang Mu (14 Chapters) with Appendix

Qing Dynasty

Containing 8 volumes in 1 case, this edition was printed by Tian De Tang in the Qing Dynasty. *Ji Yin Gang Mu* (a book on gynaecology and obstetrics) was compiled by Wu Zhiwang in the Ming Dynasty and Wang Qi in the Qing Dynasty. The books were allocated from the Library of Shaanxi University of Chinese Medicine and is still well preserved.

Preserved in Shaanxi Museum of Medical History

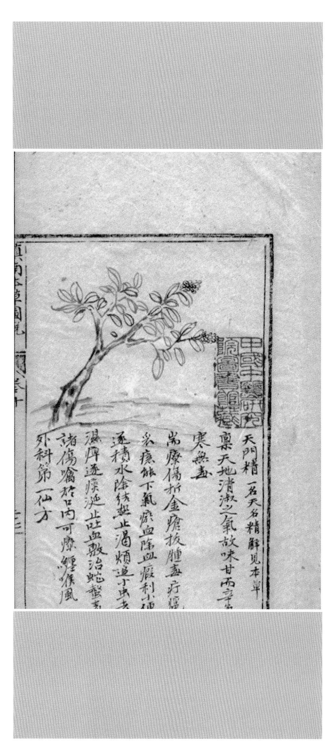

《滇南本草》

清

清代云南木刻本。成书于 1436 年。3 卷。明代兰茂纂订。本书因记述云南地区药物，故以"滇南"名书。此本收药 278 种，分为草、菜、鸟、兽、虫 5 部，各药次第述其药名、性味、功效、主治、附方，个别药物兼述其生态及形态。书中记录云南众多少数民族习用药物及用药经验，且糅合汉药部分理论，为一部独具特色的古代地方本草。

中国中医科学院图书馆藏

Dian Nan Ben Cao

Qing Dynasty

The book is the Yunnan wood-block edition. The book *Dian Nan Ben Cao* (Materia Medica in Diannan) was compiled by Lan Mao in the Ming Dynasty and finished in 1436. Containing 3 chapters, it records 278 kinds of medicine, in five categories of grass, greens, birds, beasts and insects, including the name, property, flavor, efficacy, indication, affixed prescription, and sometimes the environment and appearance. The book describes many conventional drugs and usage experiences of ethnic minorities in Yunnan Province (also called Diannan), and borrows some Chinese medicine theory, which makes it a unique localized materia medica in ancient China.

Preserved in Library of China Academy of Chinese Medical Sciences

不可近大人骨間寒熱又殺蟲毒○角主
療夢寐洩精○齒小兒五驚十二癇身熱
便溺血養精神定魂魄安五臟○白龍骨
滿四肢痿枯汗出夜卧自驚惠怒伏氣在
心下不得喘息腸癰內疽陰蝕止汗縮小
輕身通神明延年神農本經骨療心腹煩
下結氣不能喘息諸痙殺精物○角久服
驚癇○齒主小兒大人驚癇癲疾狂走心
 以上朱字

龍骨 出神農 主心腹鬼疰精物老魅欬逆
 本經
洩痢膿血女子漏下癥瘕堅結小兒熱氣

龍

《本草品汇精要》书影

清

图为清抄本。药书。明太医院集体编撰。42 卷。成书于 1505 年。本书是在《证类本草》一书基础上
改编修补而成，共收药物 1815 种。对药物的采制应用的叙述比较细致。所绘彩色药图也较逼真，但其
文字部多系抄录古书，个人发挥不多，1700 年清太医院又补撰《本草品汇精要续集》10 卷，主要根据
《本草纲目》等书增补 990 种。

日本大冢恭男藏

Book Photograph of *Ben Cao Pin Hui Jing Yao*

Qing Dynasty

Ben Cao Pin Hui Jing Yao (Concise Compilation of Herbal Foundation) is a 42-chapter medical book which is a collective compilation by the Imperial Hospital of the Ming Dynasty in 1505. Based on another book, *Zheng Lei Ben Cao*, this book contains 1,815 kinds of herbs with detailed descriptions of their gathering, decocting and application methods as well as vivid color paintings, while the content was mostly exceptions from other books without much addition. In 1700, the Imperial Hospital of the Qing Dynasty compiled another 10 chapters in the book *Ben Cao Pin Hui Jing Yao Xu Ji* (supplement to essential herb collections), which added 990 new items according to *Ben Cao Gang Mu* (Compendium of Materia Medica).

Collected by Otsuka Yasuo,Japan

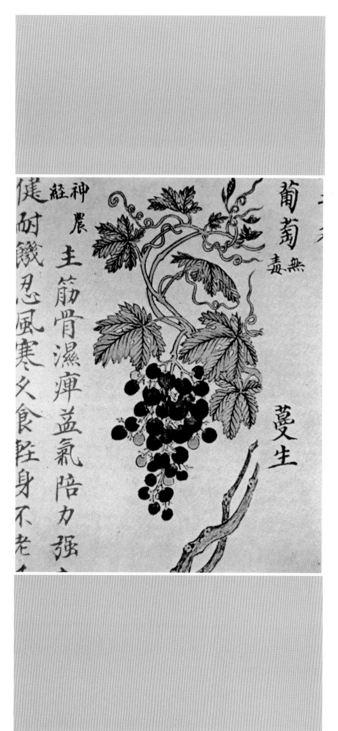

《本草品汇精要》书影

清

图为清康熙摹绘本。明代太医院院判刘文泰等奉命撰修。42 卷。全书共收载药物 1815 种，原书有王世昌等 8 名画师所绘的 1358 幅五彩工笔药图，甚为精美。原书编成后因故未得刊行而藏于内府。

罗马国立中央图书馆藏

Book Photograph of *Ben Cao Pin Hui Jing Yao*

Qing Dynasty

The book is the edition of isograph in the reign of Emperor Kangxi. *Ben Cao Pin Hui Jing Yao* (Concise Compilation of Herbal Foundation) was compiled by the Imperial Hospital official Liu Wentai and other people in the Ming Dynasty under the order of Emperor Kangxi. Containing 42 chapters, the book recorded 1,815 kinds of medicines. The original book also has 1,358 exquisite colorful paintings about medicine in elaborate style by Wang Shichang and other seven artists. The book was not published after completion and it was then preserved in the imperial storehouse.

Preserved in National Central Library of Rome

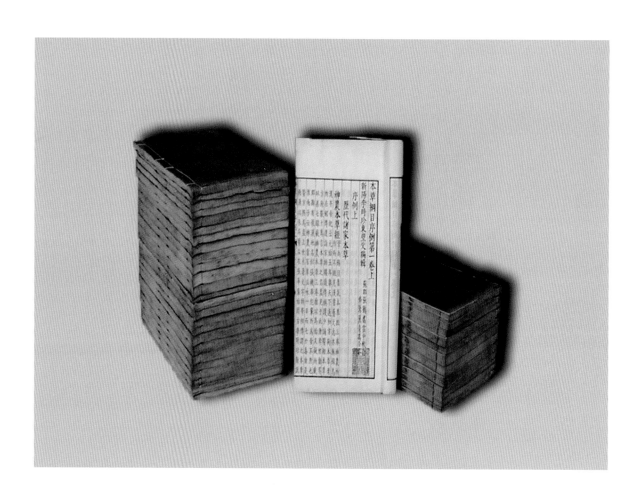

《本草纲目》

清

纵 29.3 厘米，横 19 厘米

雕版线装，清顺治十五年（1658）张朝璘刻本。保存基本完整，纸张泛黄，局部磨损。

中华医学会 / 上海中医药大学医史博物馆藏

Ben Cao Gang Mu

Qing Dynasty

Vertical Length 29.3 cm/ Horizontal Length 19 cm

This collection of *Ben Cao Gang Mu* (Compendium of Materia Medica) is the thread-binding edition and block-printed by Zhang Chaolin in 1658. The books are basically in complete condition, with yellow discoloration of the paper and the worn-out parts.

Preserved in Chinese Medical Association/ Museum of Chinese Medicine, Shanghai University of Traditional Chinese Medicine

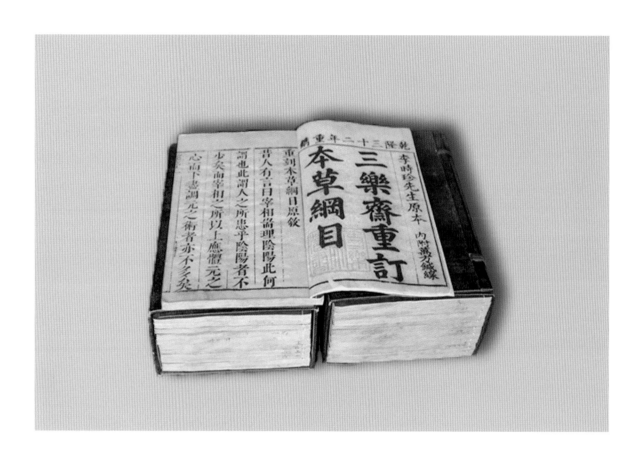

《本草纲目》五十二卷，卷首一卷，附图两卷

清

清代乾隆三十二年（1767）三乐斋校刻本。明代李时珍著，3 函 48 册。附《万方针》8 卷、《濒湖脉学》、《奇经八脉考》、《脉诀考证》。缺卷二十、二十一、二十四至三十七、三十八、四十九、五十上等，北京市中国书店选购。

陕西医史博物馆藏

Ben Cao Gang Mu (52 Chapters plus Preface and Diagrams)

Qing Dynasty

This collection is the edition proofread and block-printed by San Le Zhai in 1767, containing 48 volumes in 3 cases. *Ben Cao Gang Mu* (Compendium of Materia Medica) was written by Li Shizhen in the Ming Dynasty. This set of books also included 8 chapters of *Wan Fang Zhen* (a set of reference books that helped to find traditional Chinese medicine for specific illnesses) as well as *Bin Hu Mai Xue*, *Qi Jing Ba Mai Kao* and *Mai Jue Kao Zheng*, which are books illustrating the knowledge of sphygmology. The 20th, 21st, 24th to 37th, 38th, 49th and the 50th chapters are lost. They were purchased from the China Bookstore of Beijing.

Preserved in Shaanxi Museum of Medical History

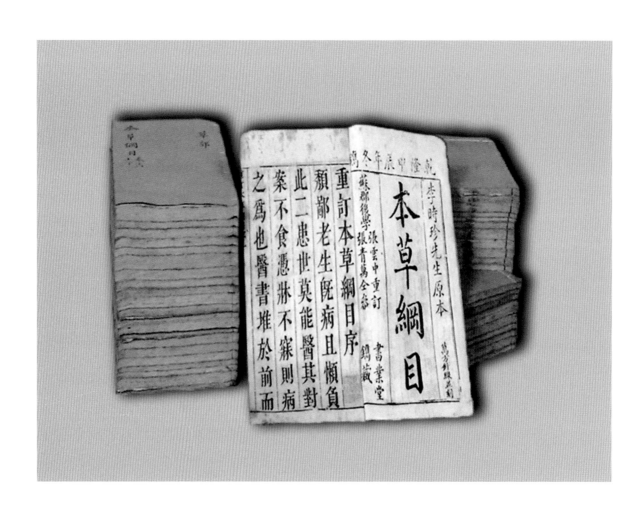

《本草纲目》

清

纵 25 厘米，横 15.8 厘米

雕版线装，清乾隆四十九年甲辰年（1784）刻本，共 43 册，与《万方针线》并刻。保存基本完整，纸张泛黄，局部磨损。

中华医学会 / 上海中医药大学医史博物馆藏

Ben Cao Gang Mu

Qing Dynasty

Vertical Length 25 cm/ Horizontal Length 15.8 cm

This collection of *Ben Cao Gang Mu* (Compendium of Materia Medica) is the thread-binding edition and block-printed in 1784. Containing 43 volumes, these books were printed together with *Wan Fang Zhen Xian* (a set of reference books that helped to find traditional Chinese medicine for specific illnesses). The books are basically well preserved with yellow discoloration and partial paper abrasion.

Preserved in Chinese Medical Association/ Museum of Chinese Medicine, Shanghai University of Traditional Chinese Medicine

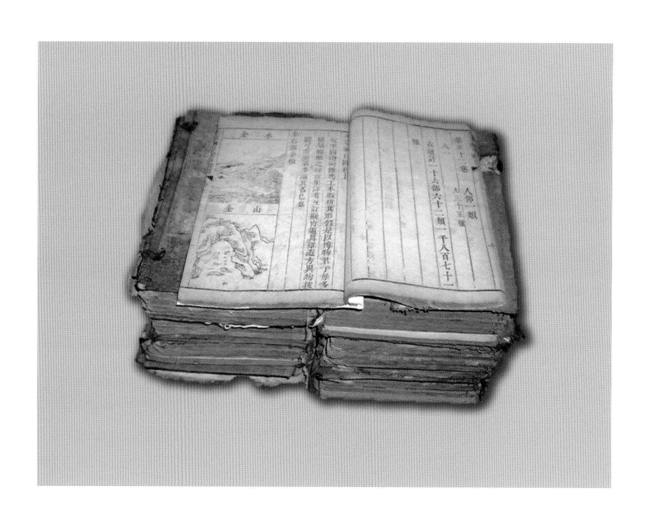

《本草纲目》五十二卷

清

清乾隆四十九年甲辰（1785）刊本，书业堂刻本。明代李时珍著，7 函 42 册。保存完整。陕西中医药大学图书馆调拨。

陕西医史博物馆藏

Ben Cao Gang Mu (52 Chapters)

Qing Dynasty

Composed of 42 volumes in 7 cases, these books are the edition proofread in 1785 and block-printed by Shu Ye Tang. *Ben Cao Gang Mu* (Compendium of Materia Medica) was written by Li Shizhen in the Ming Dynasty. The books were allocated from the Library of Shaanxi University of Chinese Medicine and are still complete.

Preserved in Shaanxi Museum of Medical History

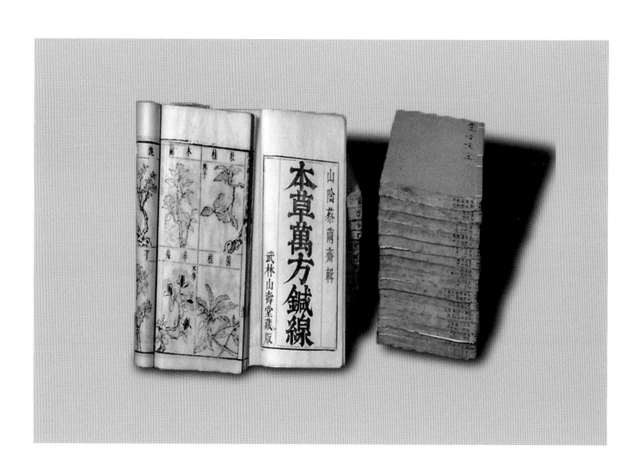

《本草万方针线》

清

纵 26.2 厘米，横 16.7 厘米

武林山寿堂藏版，山阴蔡烈先辑。全书共 30 册，雕版线装。保存基本完整，纸张泛黄，局部磨损。

中华医学会 / 上海中医药大学医史博物馆藏

Ben Cao Wan Fang Zhen Xian

Qing Dynasty

Vertical Length 26.2 cm/ Horizontal Length 16.7 cm

Ben Cao Wan Fang Zhen Xian is a set of reference books that helped to find traditional Chinese medicine for specific illnesses. This collection is the edition compiled by Cai Leixian in Shanyin County, preserved by Shan Shou Tang in Wulin County. It has 30 volumes, assembled by traditional thread binding method. The books are basically well preserved with yellow discoloration and partial paper abrasion.

Preserved in Chinese Medical Association/ Museum of Chinese Medicine, Shanghai University of Traditional Chinese Medicine

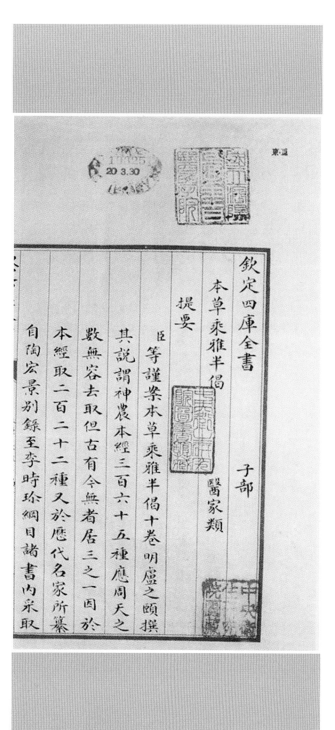

《四库全书》"子部·医家类"书

清

影抄文渊阁本。成书于乾隆五十二年(1787)。《四库全书》系清代官修的一部大型丛书，由永瑢、纪昀、陆费墀等负责编纂。本书在子部中收入了大量清代以前的医药古籍，编为医家类，此为其中《本草乘雅半偈》一书之书影。

中国中医科学院图书馆藏

Medial Category of *Si Ku Quan Shu*

Qing Dynasty

This is the edition from Wen Yuan Ge, the imperial library in the Qing Dynasty in the 52nd year of the reign of Emperor Qianlong (1787). *Si Ku Quan Shu* (Complete Library in Four Branches of Literature) was a multi-volume series of works compiled by officials in the Qing Dynasty such as Yong Rong, Ji Xian, Lu Feichi and so on. The compliers set up a special category to include a large number of medical works written before the Qing Dynasty. The picture was a book photograph of *Ben Cao Cheng Ya Ban Ji*, a medical book about the use of traditional Chinese herbal medicine.

Preserved in Library of China Academy of Chinese Medical Sciences

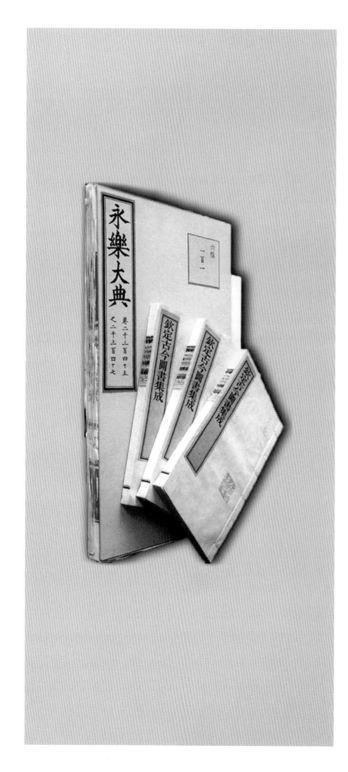

《古今图书集成·医部全录》书影

清

武英殿版。清代陈梦雷等编辑。520 卷。本书搜罗较广，收医学文献 120 余种，多标明出处。按内容分门别类，按时代先后罗列各家论述，是一部规模较大的中医学类书。

中国中医科学院图书馆藏

Book Photograph of *Gu Jin Tu Shu Ji Cheng* (Medical Part)

Qing Dynasty

The book is the edition of Wu Ying Dian. *Gu Jin Tu Shu Ji Cheng* (Collection of Ancient and Modern Books) was compiled by Chen Menglei in the Qing Dynasty. The 520-chapter book collected more than 120 categories of medical literature, most of which has its own reference. As a large-scale medical book, its content was categorized and the works of various schools were listed chronologically.

Preserved in Library of China Academy of Chinese Medical Sciences

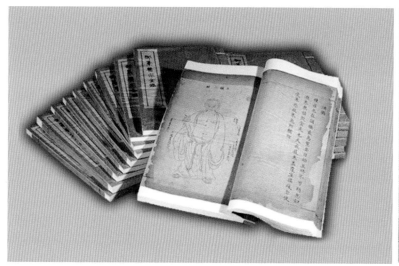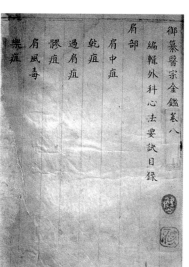

《御纂医宗金鉴》书影

清

清原稿本。成书于乾隆七年 (1742)。清太医院判吴谦等奉命编修。90 卷，收书 15 种。此书叙述简明，并多为歌诀体裁，是我国古代医学丛书中比较完备而实用的一种。图为该书《外科心法要诀》定稿本之一部分。

中国医史博物馆藏

Book Photograph of *Yu Zuan Yi Zong Jin Jian*

Qing Dynasty

The book is the original edition in the Qing Dynasty. *Yi Zong Jin Jian* (literally known as *The Golden Mirror of Medicine*) was a medical textbook complied by Imperial Hospital official Wu Qian and other people under the order of the Emperor and finally finished in the 7th year of the reign of Emperor Qianlong (1742). The compliers had collected 15 categories of books, which were arranged into 90 chapters. The book adopted a concise illustration style and the literary form of verse. Among all the other Chinese ancient medical books, it is the relatively complete and pragmatic one. The picture shows a part of the finalized edition of *Wai Ke Xin Fa Yao Jue* (a book about the important points of surgery).

Preserved in Chinese Medical History Museum

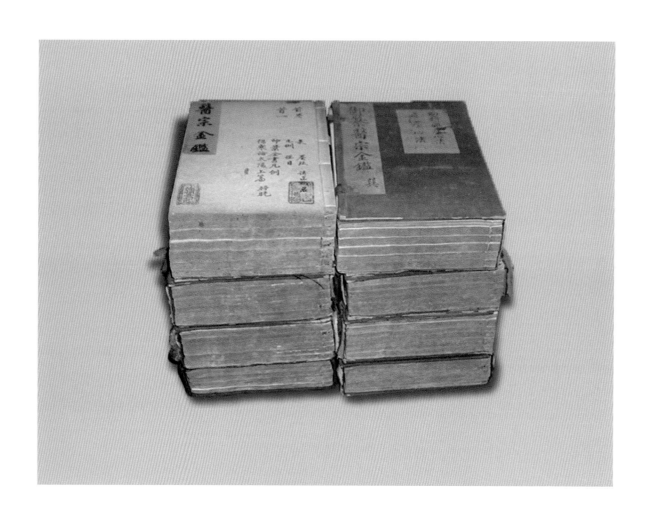

《御纂医宗金鉴》

清

清德顺堂刻本。清代吴谦等编修。8 函 48 册。子目共收医书 15 种。保存完整。北京市中国书店选购。

陕西医史博物馆藏

Yu Zuan Yi Zong Jin Jian

Qing Dynasty

The book is the block-printed edition of De Shun Tang. This collection of *Yu Zuan Yi Zong Jin Jian* (the Emperor commissioned medical book) was compiled by Wu Qian and other people in the Qing Dynasty. It has 48 volumes in 8 cases, collecting 15 kinds of medical works. The books were purchased from the China Bookstore of Beijing and are still complete.

Preserved in Shaanxi Museum of Medical History

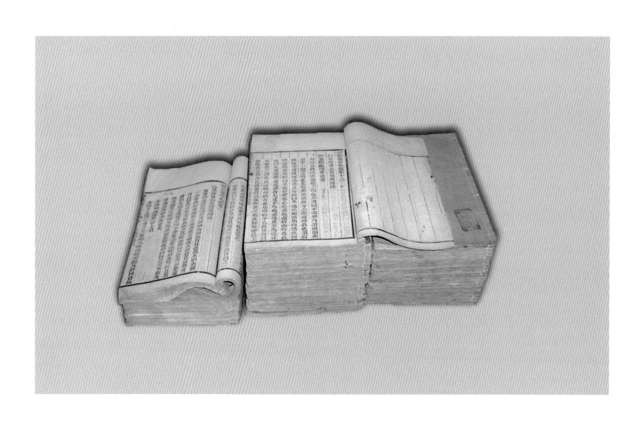

《御纂医宗金鉴》

清

清代吴谦等编修。46 册。封面题："御纂医宗金鉴"，子目共收医书 15 种，匹配本。保存完整。陕西中医药大学图书馆调拨。

陕西医史博物馆藏

Yu Zuan Yi Zong Jin Jian

Qing Dynasty

This collection of *Yu Zuan Yi Zong Jin Jian* (the Emperor commissioned medical book) was compiled by Wu Qian and other people in the Qing Dynasty. It has 46 volumes. The book's cover was titled "Yu Zuan Yi Zong Jin Jian", literally known as "the book was complied in accordance with the Emperor's commission and was used as a textbook for the Imperial Academy of Medicine". The series collected 15 categories of medical works. The books shown in the picture were the back-up edition of the original. These books were allocated from the Library of Shaanxi University of Chinese Medicine and are still complete.

Preserved in Shaanxi Museum of Medical History

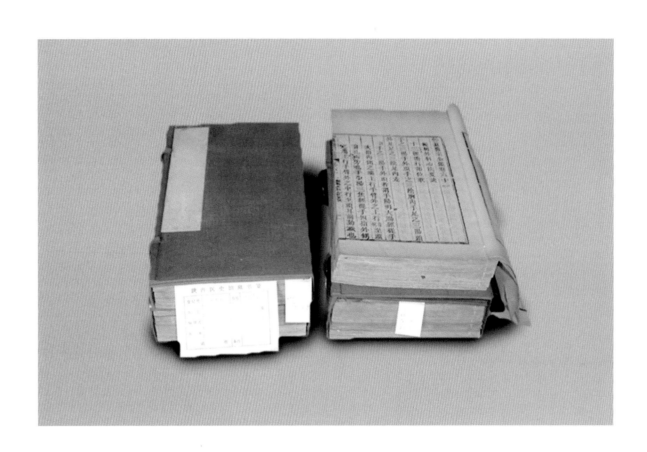

《御纂医宗金鉴》

清

版本不清，6 函 39 册。子目共有医书 15 种。不全。陕西中医药大学图书馆调拨。

陕西医史博物馆藏

Yu Zuan Yi Zong Jin Jian

Qing Dynasty

The edition of the books is not clear. This collection of *Yu Zuan Yi Zong Jin Jian* (the Emperor commissioned medical book) has 39 volumes in 6 cases. It collected 15 categories of medical works. These books were allocated from the Library of Shaanxi University of Chinese Medicine and are already incomplete.

Preserved in Shaanxi Museum of Medical History

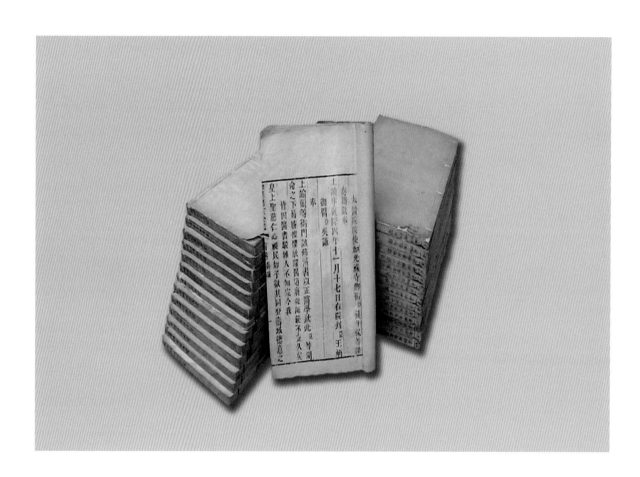

《医宗金鉴》

清

纵 24.2 厘米，横 15.2 厘米

清代吴谦等编修。全书共 90 卷，分 15 个部分，采集了自春秋战国至明清历代医著精华，内容丰富，是一部大型综合性医书。原刻本为 60 卷 30 册，为线装雕版清刻本，现藏有缺。保存基本完整，纸张泛黄，局部磨损。

中华医学会 / 上海中医药大学医史博物馆藏

Yi Zong Jin Jian

Qing Dynasty

Vertical Length 24.2 cm/ Horizontal Length 15.2 cm

Yi Zong Jin Jian, compiled by Wu Qian and other people in the Qing Dynasty, contains 90 chapters in 15 categories. This large-scale comprehensive medical series absorbed the essence of the abundant medical works dating from the Warring States Period to the Ming and Qing Dynasties. The original block-printed edition had 60 chapters in 30 volumes, which was the thread-binding edition engraved in the Qing Dynasty. The current preserved edition in the museum is not complete. The books are basically well preserved with yellow discolouration and partial paper abrasion.

Preserved in Chinese Medical Association/ Museum of Chinese Medicine, Shanghai University of Traditional Chinese Medicine

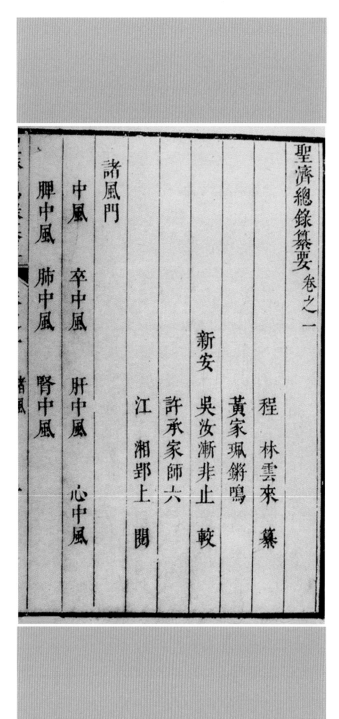

《圣济总录纂要》书影

清

康熙辛酉（1681）广陵黄绮堂刻本。《圣济总录》原系北宋政和年间（1111—1117）由宋徽宗主持编纂。全书 200 卷，包括临证各科及养生、杂治等，分为 66 门。每门首列论说，次列各种病症，凡病因、病理、方药、炮制、服法、禁忌等都有说明。后清初医学家程林对其删繁就简，摄其要旨，编为《圣济总录纂要》26 卷，此为其书影。

中国中医科学院图书馆藏

Book Photograph of *Sheng Ji Zong Lu Zuan Yao*

Qing Dynasty

The picture shows the edition of *Sheng Ji Zong Lu Zuan Yao* printed by Huang Qi Tang in Guangling County in 1681. The original book, *Sheng Ji Zong Lu*, is a medical book about different clinical subjects, health maintenance and difficult miscellaneous diseases compiled under the commission of Emperor Huizong of the Song Dynasty during 1111–1117. Containing 200 chapters and 66 categories, the book starts each category with an introduction, followed by the specific disease, with elaboration of its etiology, pathology, prescription, the way of processing, the medicine usage, contraindication and so on. In the early Qing Dynasty, a doctor named Cheng Lin simplified the original work into *Sheng Ji Zong Lu Zuan Yao* (Zuan Yao meaning major points), which has only 26 chapters.

Preserved in Library of China Academy of Chinese Medical Sciences

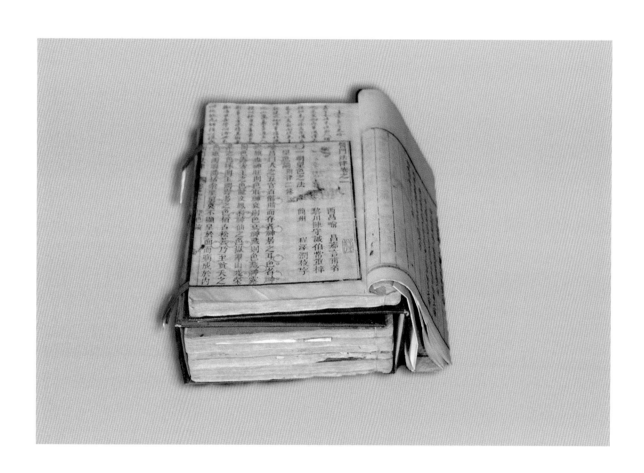

《医门法律》六卷

清

清乾隆三十年（1765），黎川陈氏集思堂刻本。清代喻昌撰。1函6册。保存完整。陕西中医药大学图书馆调拨。

陕西医史博物馆藏

Yi Men Fa Lü (6 Chapters)

Qing Dynasty

Yi Men Fa Lü is a medical book written by Yu Chang in the Qing Dynasty. It has 6 volumes in 1 case. The edition shown in the picture was printed in 1765 by Ji Si Tang, originally owned by Chen in Lichuan County, Jiangxi Province. The books were allocated from the Library of Shaanxi University of Chinese Medicine and is still complete.

Preserved in Shaanxi Museum of Medical History

溫熱論

古吳葉　桂天士甫箸　皖南建德周學海注

溫熱論從唐本

溫邪上受首先犯肺逆傳心胞　時感者雲日風溫濕溫之邪從口鼻而入者非世上邪從口鼻而入莫上人之

者不受也按傷寒若從毛竅而入温時伏寒從口鼻有汗法亦本寒素盛熱二者亦皆互上受二字卽盡內從表裏邪氣而在入遂入

不受也日上受若從毛竅而入温時伏寒從少陰又語一以全按傷寒若春温之由冬時伏寒從口鼻而入其實二者亦病從口鼻

何以治法中鼻有汗法亦不察文上甚一受也若總以從毛竅合一在入遂入

似者馮多定人案矣其焦淫熱而本實以入二者

義上論肺主氣屬衛心主血屬營辨營衛氣血雖與傷寒同

若論治法則與傷寒大異蓋傷寒之邪留戀在表然後

化熱入裏溫邪則化熱最速未傳心胞邪尙在肺肺合

皮毛而主氣故云在表初用辛涼輕劑挾風加薄荷牛

《温热论》书影

清

《周氏医学丛书》本。本书系清代叶天士讲授，其门人顾景文、华岫云等据笔记整理而成。1卷。重点揭示温热病的一般传变规律，发前人所未发；其温热病的辨证论治纲领，补前代典籍所未备。

中国中医科学院图书馆藏

Book Photograph of *Wen Re Lun*

Qing Dynasty

Included in *Zhou Shi Yi Xue Cong Shu* (series of medical books written by the Zhou's), it was originally the teaching materials of a doctor named Ye Tianshi in the Qing Dynasty and was compiled into a medical work by his disciples Gu Jingwen, Hua Xiuyun and so on. Containing only 1 chapter, it discussed patterns of transmission and changing of epidemic febrile diseases, as well as phenomena regarding this disease that was not noticed by predecessors. The guiding principle of this book for treatment was based on syndrome differentiation regarding epidemic febrile diseases, which serves as the supplement to the ancient books and records.

Preserved in Library of China Academy of Chinese Medical Sciences

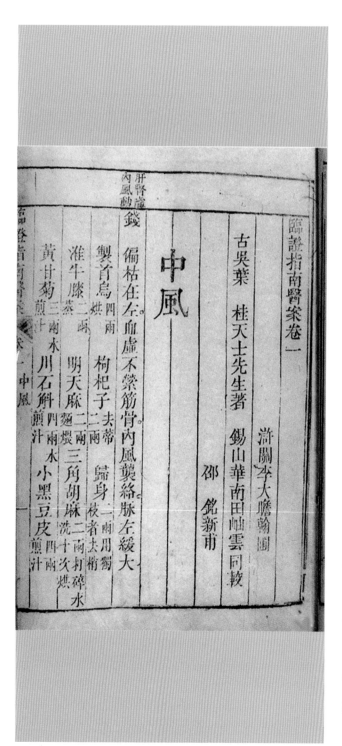

《临证指南医案》书影

清

乾隆三十三年 (1768) 刊本。本书系叶天士临证之医案，由其门人华岫云等辑成刊行。全书 10 卷，分 90 篇，叶氏临证经验主要集中于本书。叶天士 (1667—1746)，名桂，号香岩，江苏吴县 (今苏州) 人，清代医家。其对温热病的诊治有很大贡献。

Book Photograph of *Lin Zheng Zhi Nan Yi An*

Qing Dynasty

The book is the edition in 1768. *Lin Zheng Zhi Nan Yi An* was originally the clinical records of a doctor named Ye Tianshi and was compiled and published as a medical book by his disciples Hua Xiuyun and so on. It has 10 chapters and 90 articles. Ye Tianshi (1667–1746, given name Gui and pseudonym Xiangyan), was a doctor in the Qing Dynasty and was born in Wuxian County (now Suzhou City) in Jiangsu Province. Ye Tianshi made a significant contribution to the diagnosis and treatment of epidemic febrile diseases.

Preserved in Library of China Academy of Chinese Medical Sciences

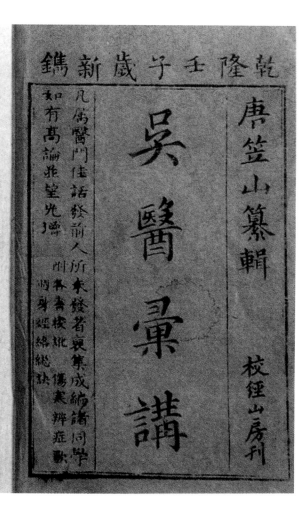

《吴医汇讲》书影

清

乾隆壬子年（1792）校经山房刊本。清代唐大烈编辑，系我国最早具备医学刊物性质的著作，共出版11卷。
因由江浙地区医家供稿故名。内容大多是学术理论的探讨文章，丰富多彩。图为其创刊号。

上海中医药博物馆藏

Book Photograph of *Wu Yi Hui Jiang*

Qing Dynasty

This edition was printed by Jiao Jing Shan Fang,
during the reign of Emperor Qianlong (1792). *Wu
Yi Hui Jiang*, compiled by Tang Dalie in the Qing
Dynasty, was China's earliest medical journal,
11 chapters of which had been published. It is
the collection of the articles written by doctors
in Jiangsu and Zhejiang Provinces. That is how
the book got its name. The book is mainly about
theoretical discussion on various topics. The
picture is its debut issue.

Preserved in Shanghai Museum of Traditional
Chinese Medicine

《温病条辨》书影

清

嘉庆十八年癸酉（1813）刊本。清代医家吴瑭撰。6卷。成书于嘉庆三年（1798）。书中对温热病的病机、辨证、论治、方药等均有精辟论述。吴瑭（1758—1836），字鞠通，江苏淮阴人。

中国中医科学院图书馆藏

Book Photograph of *Wen Bing Tiao Bian*

Qing Dynasty

The book is the block-printed edition in 1813. *Wen Bing Tiao Bian* (Identification of Warm Diseases) was written by a doctor named Wu Tang in the Qing Dynasty and completed in 1798. The six-chapter book made an incisive exposition of the etiology, syndrome differentiation, treatment variation and prescription regarding epidemic febrile disease. Wu Tang (1758–1836), with a courtesy name as Jutong, was born in Huaiyin County, Jiangsu Province.

Preserved in Library of China Academy of Chinese Medical Sciences

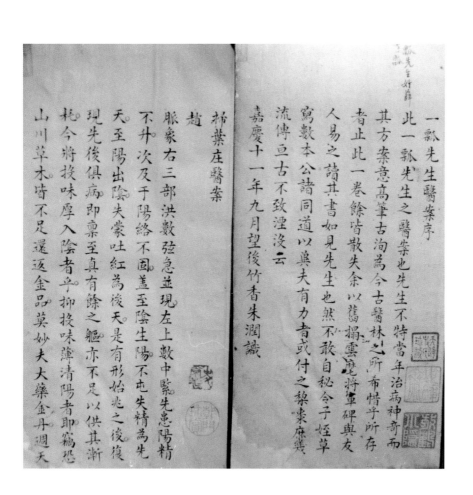

《扫叶庄医案》书影

清

嘉庆十一年（1806）朱润转录本。薛雪撰。1卷。收存薛氏医案150例，为其后本书各印本的祖本。
曾为清代医家陆懋修所珍藏。

史常永供稿

Book Photograph of *Sao Ye Zhuang Yi An*

Qing Dynasty

This edition was transcribed by Zhu Run in 1806, and was the origin of other reprinted editions. *Sao Ye Zhuang Yi An* (Medical Cases of Saoyezhuang) was written by Xue Xue. Containing only one chapter, it collected 150 clinical cases treated by the author. The book was once a private collection of a famous doctor in the Qing Dynasty named Lu Maoxiu.

Provided by Shi Changyong

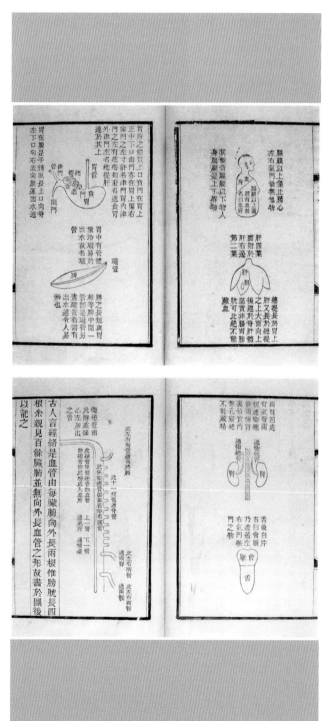

《医林改错》书影

清

光绪二十三年 (1897) 鄂藩使署校刊本。王清任著。分上、下卷。成书于道光十年 (1830)。上卷较为详细地论述了脏腑的生理解剖，敢于纠正古代医书记载的某些错误，但亦有误改之处。附有数幅脏腑改错图。下卷阐述其逐瘀活血、补气活血等理论和治法，并论述了半身不遂等病症的诊治。自订方剂 30 余首。图为其脏腑改错图书影 2 幅。

中国中医科学院图书馆藏

Book Photograph of *Yi Lin Gai Cuo*

Qing Dynasty

This edition was proofread by Er Fan Shi Shu (the name of an embassy) and printed in 1897. *Yi Lin Gai Cuo* (Correction of Errors of Medical Works) was written by Wang Qingren and finished in 1830. The book is divided into two parts. The first part elaborates the anatomy regarding human internal organs and points out mistakes in ancient medical works (though some of the corrections are erroneous) along with corrected drawing of these organs. The second part illustrates theories about promoting blood circulation for removing blood stasis and restoring vital energy, and also discusses the diagnosis and treatment of diseases like hemiplegia. The author invented about 30 prescriptions. The two pictures are the corrected edition of human organs in the book.

Preserved in Library of China Academy of Chinese Medical Sciences

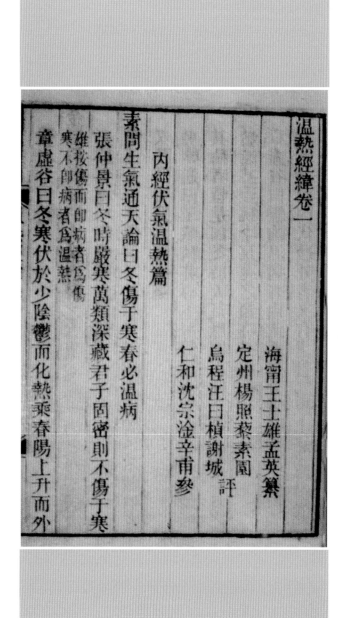

《温热经纬》书影

清

咸丰二年壬子（1852）刊本。清代王士雄撰。
5卷。成书于咸丰二年（1852）。此书以《黄
帝内经》《伤寒论》之文为经，以叶天士、
薛生白诸家之辨为纬，故名。书中收录了清
代重要温病学家叶天士、薛生白、余师愚、
陈平伯、章楠、吴鞠通、华岫云及作者本人
的学术论述，可视为清代温病学说的总汇。

中国中医科学院图书馆藏

Book Photograph of *Wen Re Jing Wei*

Qing Dynasty

The book is the edition in 1852. *Wen Re Jing Wei* (Compendium on Epidemic Febrile Diseases) was written by Wang Shixiong in the Qing Dynasty and finished in 1852. The book has 5 chapters. The main thread of the book was the articles and theories from books *Huang Di Nei Jing* and *Shang Hai Lun*, with theories of Ye Tianshi, Xue Shengbai, and other traditional medical practitioners as the supplementary, hence it got the name *Wen Re Jing Wei* (Jing means main thread; Wei means supplementary). This book included academic contributions of some important experts of seasonal febrile diseases in the Qing Dynasty, such as Ye Tianshi, Xue Shengbai, Yu Shiyu, Chen Pingbo, Zhang Nan, Wu Jutong, Hua Xiuyun, and the author himself. This book was regarded as a summary of the relevant theories in the Qing Dynasty.

Preserved in Library of China Academy of Chinese Medical Sciences

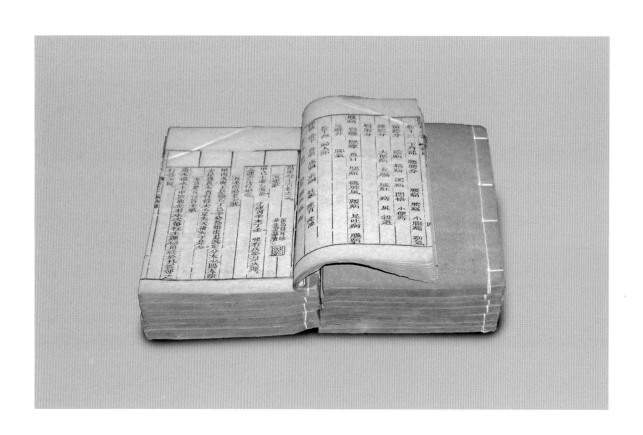

《嵩崖尊生》十五卷

清

三让堂刻本。清代景日昣撰。12 册。陕西中医药大学图书馆调拨。

陕西医史博物馆藏

Song Ya Zun Sheng (15 Chapters)

Qing Dynasty

Song Ya Zun Sheng is the block-printed edition of San Rang Tang. It was written by Jing Rizhen in the Qing Dynasty and contains 12 volumes. The books were allocated from the Library of Shaanxi University of Chinese Medicine.

Preserved in Shaanxi Museum of Medical History

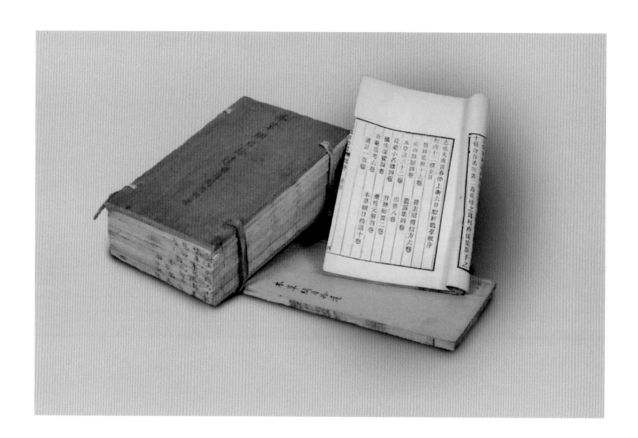

《本草纲目拾遗》

清

纵 24.2 厘米，横 14.5 厘米

《本草纲目拾遗》著者为清人赵学敏，书凡 10 卷，药分 18 部，共载药 921 种，1765—1803 年成书。

该藏本为雕版线装，版本待考。保存基本完整，纸张泛黄，局部磨损。

中华医学会 / 上海中医药大学医史博物馆藏

Ben Cao Gang Mu Shi Yi

Qing Dynasty

Vertical Length 24.2 cm/ Horizontal Length 14.5 cm

The book *Ben Cao Gang Mu Shi Yi* (Supplement to the Compendium of Materia Medica) was written by Zhao Xuemin in the Qing Dynasty during 1765–1803. The book has 10 chapters, recording 921 kinds of Chinese herbs in 18 categories. This collection is a thread-bound book by engraving. The edition remains to be verified. It is basically well preserved with yellow discoloration and regional abrasions.

Preserved in Chinese Medical Association/ Museum of Chinese Medicine, Shanghai University of Traditional Chinese Medicine

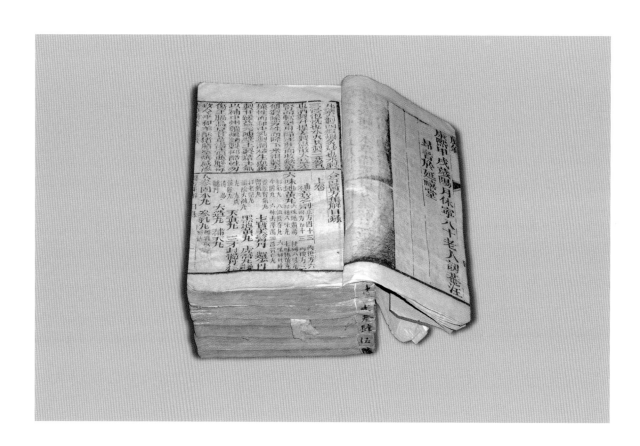

《图注本草医方合编》

清

裕德堂刻本。清代汪昂编。6 册。每页两重楼，备要、歌括在上，医方集解在下。保存完整。陕西中医药大学图书馆调拨。

陕西医史博物馆藏

Tu Zhu Ben Cao Yi Fang He Bian

Qing Dynasty

This collection is the block-printed edition of Yu De Tang. *Tu Zhu Ben Cao Yi Fang He Bian* (Illustrated Compilation of Herbal Prescriptions with Explanatory Text) was compiled by Wang Ang in the Qing Dynasty. It has 6 volumes. There are two parts in each page: the summary verses on the upper half and collection of prescriptions on the lower half. It was allocated from the Library of Shaanxi University of Chinese Medicine and is still complete.

Preserved in Shaanxi Museum of Medical History

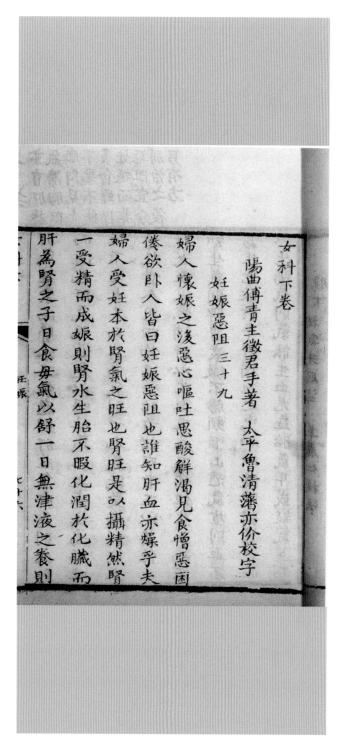

女科下卷

陽曲傅青主徵君手著 太平魯清藩亦价校字

妊娠惡阻三十九

婦人懷娠之後惡心嘔吐思酸解渴見食憎惡困

倦欲臥人皆曰妊娠惡阻也誰知肝血亦燥乎夫

婦人受妊本於腎氣之旺也腎旺是以攝精然腎

一受精而成娠則腎水生胎不暇化潤於肝化臟而

肝為腎之子日食母氣以舒一日無津液之養則

《傅青主女科》书影

清

道光七年丁亥（1827）刊本。傅山撰。2卷。
上卷收录带下、血崩、鬼胎、调经、种子等
5门38条；下卷载妊娠、小产、难产、正产、
产后诸症等5门39条。论述简明扼要，遣
方用药精当。

中国中医科学院图书馆藏

Book Photograph of *Fu Qing Zhu Nü Ke*

Qing Dynasty

This collection is the edition in 1827. *Fu Qing Zhu Nü Ke* (Fu's Obstetrics and Gynecology) was written by Fu Shan. The book was divided into 2 chapters. Chapter Ⅰ recorded 38 diseases in five categories, such as morbid leucorrhea, endometrorrhagia, stillbirth, regulating menstruation, and impregnation. Chapter Ⅱ recorded 39 diseases in five categories such as pregnancy, abortion, dystocia, regular production, and postpartum diseases, each with concise discussion and appropriate prescription. Preserved in Library of China Academy of Chinese Medical Sciences

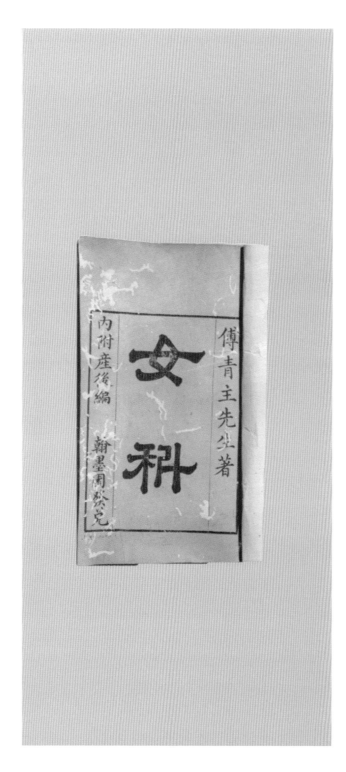

《女科》一册

清

纵 23 厘米，横 14 厘米

即《傅青主女科》，明末清初傅青主（山）撰。

其重视肝、脾、肾三脏病机，病善用气血双补、

脾胃调理之法，深受妇产科医家推崇。

广东中医药博物馆藏

Nü Ke (Volume Ⅰ)

Qing Dynasty

Vertical Length 23 cm/ Horizontal Length 14 cm

Nü Ke, namely *Fu Qing Zhu Nü Ke* (Fu's Obstetrics and Gynecology), was written by Fu Qingzhu in the late Ming and early Qing Dynasty. The author attached importance to pathogenesis of liver, spleen, and kidney. He advocated treating diseases by using Qi and blood. His treatment for regulating spleen and stomach won undivided admiration by other Chinese physicians of obstetrics and gynecology.

Preserved in Guangdong Chinese Medicine Museum

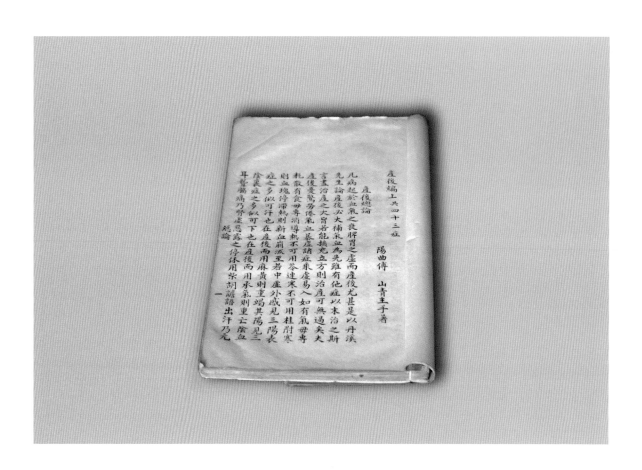

《产后编》

清

清代傅山（青主）撰。1册。抄本。

Chan Hou Bian (After Childbirth)

Qing Dynasty

The author was Fu Shan (other name Qingzhu) in the Qing Dynasty. There is only 1 volume in the book. It is a hand-copied one.

Preserved in Shaanxi Museum of Medical History

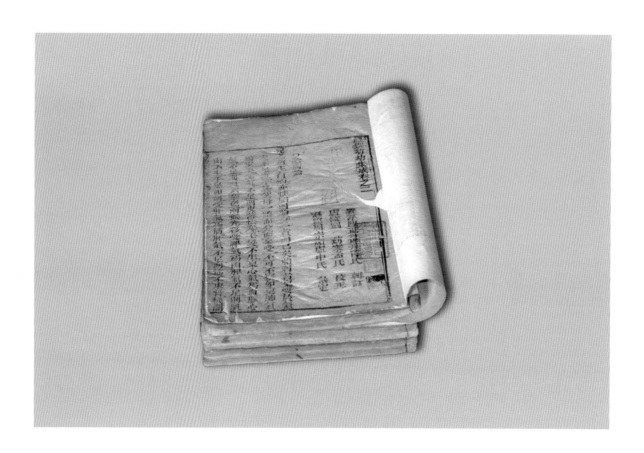

《幼幼集成》六卷

清

金裕堂刻本。清代陈复正（飞霞）编，刘襄校。6 册。保存完整。陕西中医药大学图书馆调拨。

陕西医史博物馆藏

You You Ji Cheng (6 Chapters)

Qing Dynasty

This collection is the block-printed edition of Jin Yu Tang. The book was compiled by Chen Fuzheng (other name Feixia) in the Qing Dynasty and proofread by Liu Xiang (Cai Meng). It has 6 volumes. It was allocated from the Library of Shaanxi University of Chinese Medicine and is still well-preserved.

Preserved in Shaanxi Museum of Medical History

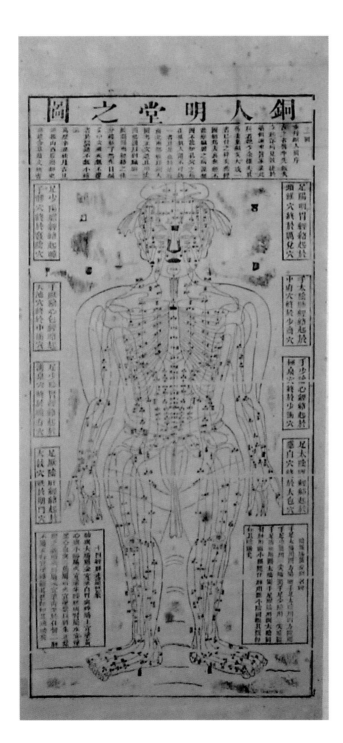

《铜人明堂之图》

清

画轴：长 144 厘米，宽 60.2 厘米

画芯：长 114.2 厘米，宽 53.3 厘米

图卷，医用图。该明堂图共四幅一组，是康熙四年渔阳林起龙复刻明万历辛丑赵含章（文炳）版本之刊印图。此幅为图一，图面画人体正面腧穴经络分布图，图上方有赵含章书"重刊铜人图序"。赵含章，名文炳，万历年间官至巡按，山西监察御史，著有《针灸大成》，绘铜人明堂图四幅。已裱成卷轴，保存基本完好。1957 年入藏。

中华医学会／上海中医药大学医史博物馆藏

Tong Ren Ming Tang Zhi Tu

Qing Dynasty

Scroll: Length 144 cm/ Width 60.2 cm

Painting: Length 114.2cm/ Width 53.3 cm

Tong Ren Ming Tang Zhi Tu is a medical chart of acupuncture and moxibustion. The whole chart consists of four pictures. It is the reprint copied by Lin Qilong in the Qing Dynasty according to Zhao Hanzhang's version in the Ming Dynasty. This is the first chart, which shows the anterior human meridian system. On the top of the chart, there are characters "Chong Kan Tong Ren Tu Xu" written by Zhao Hanzhang. Zhao Hanzhang (also known as Wenbing) was Xun An (an official title in Ming Dynasty) and was appointed as supervisory censor in Shanxi Province during the reign of Emperor Wanli. He was the author of *Zhen Jiu Da Cheng* (Integration of Acupuncture and Moxibustion) and drew four acupuncture and moxibustion charts which were made into scrolls and are well preserved. The painting was collected in 1957.

Preserved in Chinese Medical Association/ Museum of Chinese Medicine, Shanghai University of Traditional Chinese Medicine

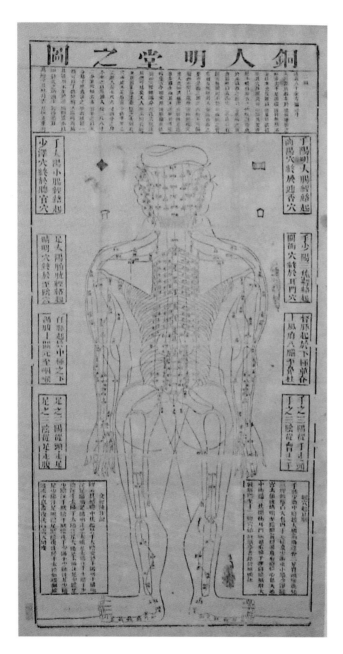

《铜人明堂之图》

清

画轴：长 144 厘米，宽 60.2 厘米

画芯：长 114.2 厘米，宽 53.3 厘米

图卷，医用图。该明堂图共四幅一组，是康熙四年渔阳林起龙复刻明万历辛丑赵含章（文炳）版本之刊印图。此幅为图二，图面画人体背面腧穴经络分布图，图上方有"孙真人千金方图经序""万历辛丑桂月吉旦校正重刊"。已裱成卷轴，保存基本完好。1957 年入藏。

中华医学会 / 上海中医药大学医史博物馆藏

Tong Ren Ming Tang Zhi Tu

Qing Dynasty

Scroll: Length 144 cm/Width 60.2 cm

Painting: Length 114.2cm/ Width 53.3 cm

Tong Ren Ming Tang Zhi Tu is a medical chart of acupuncture and moxibustion. The whole chart consists of four pictures. It is the reprint copied by Lin Qilong in the Qing Dynasty according to Zhao Hanzhang's version in the Ming Dynasty. This is the second chart, which shows the reverse human meridian system. On the top of the chart, there are characters meaning "the introductory map of *Qian Jin Fang*", as well as 12 characters meaning "this painting was reprint correction in the reign of Emperor Wanli". The painting was made into scroll and is well preserved. It was collected in 1957.

Preserved in Chinese Medical Association/ Museum of Chinese Medicine, Shanghai University of Traditional Chinese Medicine

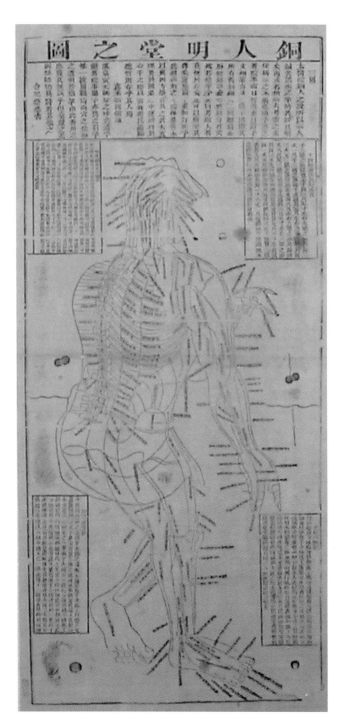

《铜人明堂之图》

清

画轴：长 144 厘米，宽 60.2 厘米

画芯：长 114.2 厘米，宽 53.3 厘米

图卷，医用图。该明堂图共四幅一组，是康熙四年渔阳林起龙复刻明万历辛丑赵含章（文炳）版本之刊印图。此幅为图三，图面画人体背面右侧腧穴经络分布图，图上方有合肥蔡悉书文。已裱成卷轴，保存基本完好。1957 年入藏。

中华医学会 / 上海中医药大学医史博物馆藏

Tong Ren Ming Tang Zhi Tu

Qing Dynasty

Scroll: Length 144 cm/ Width 60.2 cm

Painting: Length 114.2cm/ Width 53.3 cm

Tong Ren Ming Tang Zhi Tu is a medical chart of acupuncture and moxibustion. The whole chart consists of four pictures. It is the reprint copied by Lin Qilong in the Qing Dynasty according to Zhao Hanzhang's version in the Ming Dynasty. This chart is the third one, which shows the right side of the reverse human meridian system. On the top of the painting, there are characters written by Cai Xi. The chart was made into scroll and is well preserved. The painting was collected in 1957.

Preserved in Chinese Medical Association/ Museum of Chinese Medicine, Shanghai University of Traditional Chinese Medicine

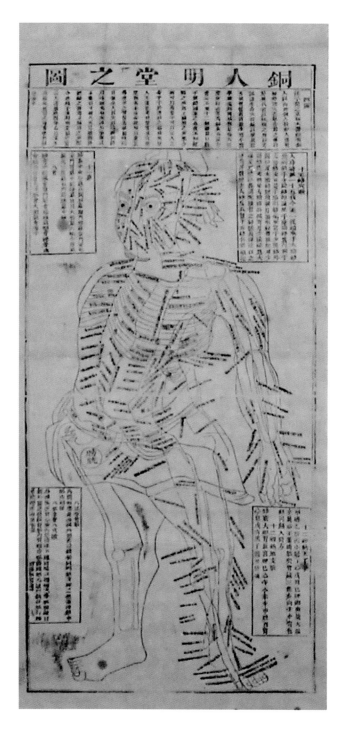

《铜人明堂之图》

清

画轴：长 144 厘米，宽 60.2 厘米

画芯：长 114.2 厘米，宽 53.3 厘米

图卷，医用图。该明堂图共四幅一组，是康熙四年渔阳林起龙复刻明万历辛丑赵含章（文炳）版本之刊印图。此幅为图四，图面画人体左侧腧穴经络分布图，图上方有渔阳林起龙撰复刻明堂图文。林起龙，字北海，清代医家，渔阳人，辑有《本草纲目必读》（1667）。已裱成卷轴，保存基本完好。1957 年入藏。

中华医学会 / 上海中医药大学医史博物馆藏

Tong Ren Ming Tang Zhi Tu

Qing Dynasty

Scroll: Length 144 cm/ Width 60.2 cm

Painting: Length 114.2cm/ Width 53.3 cm

Tong Ren Ming Tang Zhi Tu is a medical chart of acupuncture and moxibustion. The whole chart consists of four pictures. It is the reprint copied by Lin Qilong in the Qing Dynasty according to Zhao Hanzhang's version in the Ming Dynasty. This chart is the fourth one, which shows the left side of the human meridian system. On the top of it, there are characters meaning "this is re-carved copy by Lin Qilong according to the version in the Ming Dynasty". Lin Qilong, with his courtesy name Beihai, was a traditional Chinese physician in the Qing Dynasty. His hometown was Yuyang County (now in City of Beijing). He was the author of *Ben Cao Gang Mu Bi Du* (Quintessence of the Compendium of Materia Medica) (1667). The chart was made into scroll and is well preserved. The painting was collected in 1957.

Preserved in Chinese Medical Association/ Museum of Chinese Medicine, Shanghai University of Traditional Chinese Medicine

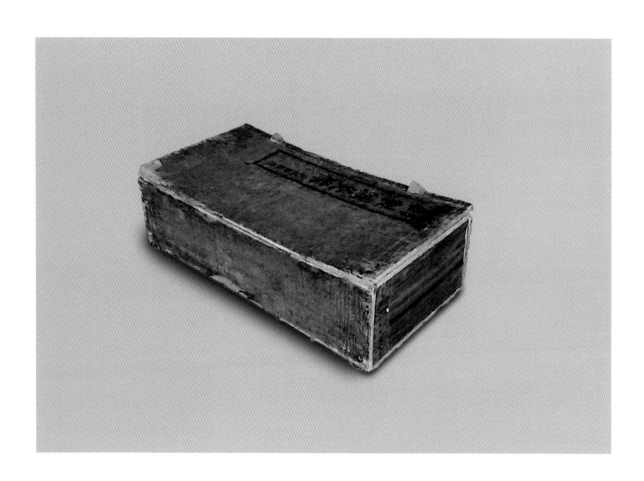

针灸铜人锦盒

清

长 29.5 厘米，宽 14 厘米，高 58 厘米

该藏是我馆收藏的清乾隆针灸铜人的外包装锦盒。该针灸铜人与盒是乾隆时御赐修纂《医宗金鉴》正蓝旗人福海之物。盒内盖和底载有御制针灸铜人一文。另附御制针灸像重修记一册，系清光绪癸卯年福海九世孙振声所纂。长方形，用于装帧。纸盒面翘卷，破损较重，纸面泛黄，字迹局部脱落，御玺印记模糊不清。

中华医学会／上海中医药大学医史博物馆藏

Brocade Box of Bronze Acupuncture Figure

Qing Dynasty

Length 29.5 cm / Width 14 cm / Height 58 cm

This collection is the brocade box for outer packing of the bronze acupuncture figure in the reign of Emperor Qianlong in the Qing Dynasty. Both the bronze acupuncture figure and the box were possessed by nobility Fu Hai, who was also the owner of Emperor Qianlong commissioned version of *Yi Zong Jin Jian*, a medical book. There are articles about the imperial bronze acupuncture figure on both the inner cap and the bottom of the box. There was also a book recording the recast of the acupuncture figure, which was written by Zhen Sheng, the ninth generation offspring of Fu Hai during the reign of Emperor Guangxu in the Qing Dynasty. This collection is oblong, easy for binding and layout. The surface of the box is curl and seriously damaged. The paper has yellow discoloration with partial characters fading off. The royal seal's signet is blurred.

Preserved in Chinese Medical Association/ Museum of Chinese Medicine, Shanghai University of Traditional Chinese Medicine

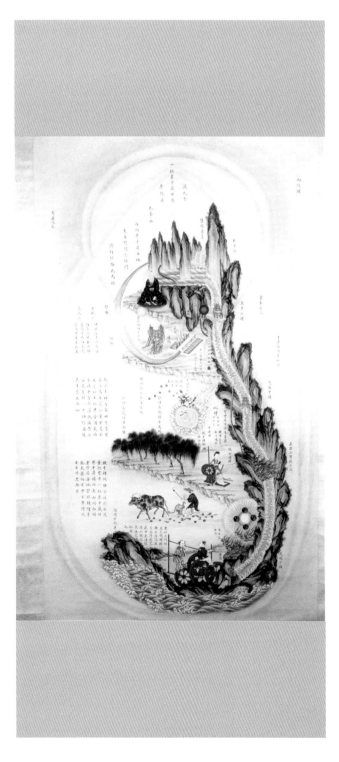

《内景图》

清

纵 168 厘米，横 97 厘米

此图由清宫如意馆绘制，为气功内功图解。内景，即人体内部精神变化之意，古代气功学家认为人体内为一小宇宙，以此比拟其生理、解剖关系，绘成此图，因名为内景图。其是练功者的重要参考图录。

中国医史博物馆藏

Nei Jing Tu

Qing Dynasty

Vertical Length 168 cm/ Horizontal Length 97 cm

This collection of *Nei Jing Tu* (Interior Figure) was drawn by Ru Yi Guan, the Imperial Gallery, to diagrammatize the spiritual change of interior body. Ancient Qigong experts thought that the internal force of human body was a microcosm. The painter took this metaphor to describe the relationship between anatomy and physiology. That is how this picture came into being and got its name. It was an important reference for Qigong practitioners.

Preserved in Chinese Medical History Museum

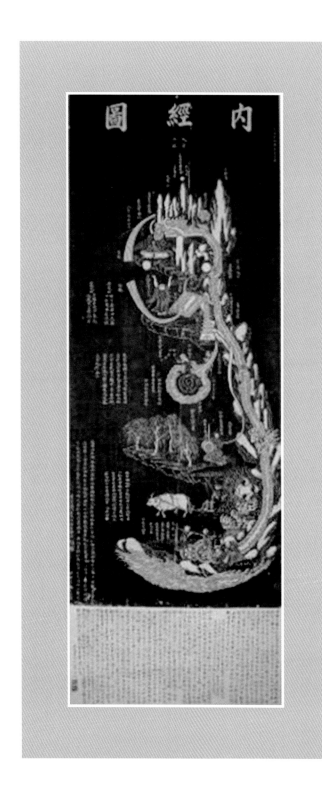

《道藏内景图》木刻拓本

清

纵 127 厘米，横 53 厘米

此图为道教练功图。道教养生偏重精神修养，以静生为入门之学，旧传得道者，能收视敛听，内观返照，却病延年，最者可成仙。本图即经静坐原理，按人体生理作用，以类比附机械构造而成的生理示意图，所绘各部男女老幼人物隐喻生长变化代谢循环，为究凡道家养生之术。版藏燕京西部白云观，此为其拓本。

广东中医药博物馆藏

Wood Carving Rubbing of *Taoist Interior Figure*

Qing Dynasty

Vertical Length 127cm / Horizontal Length 53 cm

This picture is a practicing figure of Taoism. The theory of preserving one's health in Taoism focuses on spiritual practices, taking "Jing Sheng" (silent spiritual life style) as the entry level. One who attained the Dao by focusing on the inner feeling could achieve longevity. The one who absorbed the essence could be immortal. This picture took "Jing Jing Zuo" as the principle and followed the function of human physiology. It was a schematic diagram of physiology by comparing it to the mechanical composition. The figures on the picture were metaphors of the metabolic cycle during human variations. It was the method of health maintenance of Taoism. The authentic work was preserved in the Bai Yun Guan in west Beijing. This collection is the rubbing of it.

Preserved in Guangdong Chinese Medicine Museum

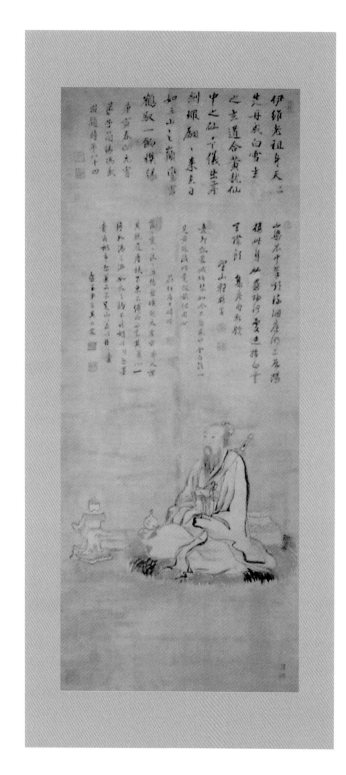

蔡嘉绘《纯阳炼丹图》

清

卷轴：长 199.5 厘米，宽 53.6 厘米

画芯：长 97.8 厘米，宽 40 厘米

卷轴，为书画。其为蔡嘉于清乾隆三十五年
（1770）所绘（绢画），画面为吕纯阳炼丹图。
右下角有白文"蔡嘉"及朱文"雪堂"钤记，
上方有简员、冯武、程枚吉、吴汝霖等题字。
蔡嘉，清代乾隆时人，字松原，号雪堂，江
苏丹阳人，善书画，尤善青山绿水，是乾隆
年间著名画家。已裱成卷轴，绢面泛黄，画
面有损坏。1958 年入藏。

中华医学会 / 上海中医药大学医史博物馆藏

Chun Yang Lian Dan Tu by Cai Jia

Qing Dynasty

Scroll: Length 199.5 cm/ Width 53.6 cm

Painting: Length 97.8cm/ Width 40 cm

This collection of *Chun Yang Lian Dan Tu* (Figure of Chun Yang's Alchemy) was drawn by Cai Jia in the 35th year during the reign of Emperor Qianlong (1770) in the Qing Dynasty. It is a classical Chinese painting on silk showing Lü Chunyang's alchemy. At the lower right corner, there are intagliated characters "Cai Jia" and "Xue Tang" carved in relief. On the upper half, there are inscriptions made by Jian Yuan, Feng Wu, Feng Meiji, Wu Ruilin and so on. Cai Jia (courtesy name Songyuan, pseudonym Xuetang) was born in Danyang County, Jiangsu Province. As a famous painter during the reign of Emperor Qianlong, he was especially adept at landscape painting. The painting has been made into scroll and was collected in 1958. The figure was partially damaged, with yellow discoloration on the surface of the silk.

Preserved in Chinese Medical Association/ Museum of Chinese Medicine, Shanghai University of Traditional Chinese Medicine

杨法篆书《心铭》轴

清

纵 173.5 厘米，横 36 厘米

篆书。杨法篆书，为清代书坛风格独异者，受明代书家赵
凡夫草篆及清代郑谷口隶书影响，作篆融会篆、隶、草于
一炉，使篆书更富装饰性，写来笔意古雅，洒脱如行云流水。

南京市博物馆藏

Calligraphy Scroll of *Xin Ming* by Yang Fa

Qing Dynasty

Vertical Length 173.5 cm/ Horizontal Length 36 cm

There are seal characters on the scroll written by Yang Fa, who had special style in Qing Dynasty's calligraphy world. He was influenced by Zhao Fanfu's cursive seal script in the Ming Dynasty and Zheng Gukou's clerical script in the Qing Dynasty. His calligraphy is ornamental, elegant, natural and smooth by synthesizing seal script, clerical script, and cursive script as a whole.

Preserved in Nanjing Municipal Museum

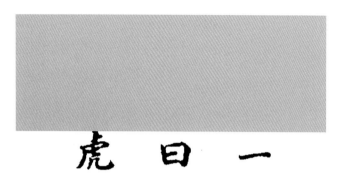

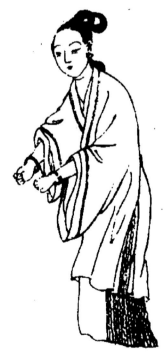

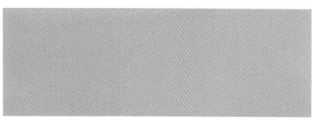

《五禽戏图谱·虎戏》

清

选自席裕康《内外功图说辑要》。此书辑录有多种古代保健养生方法的图谱，五禽戏图谱是其中之一。它是模仿虎、熊、鹿、猿、鸟五种动物的行为来锻炼身体的一种导引养生方法，为东汉名医华佗在前人的基础上创编而成。此为五禽戏之一——虎戏。

中国国家图书馆藏

Wu Qin Xi Tu Pu-Tiger Exercises

Qing Dynasty

The picture was selected from *Nei Wai Gong Tu Shuo Ji Yao* (Graphic Summary of Exercises to Benefit Inner Organs, Muscle and Bone) compiled by Xi Yukang. This book includes many kinds of pictures of health maintenance in ancient times. *Wu Qin Xi Tu Pu* (Atlas of Five-Animal Exercises) is one of them, showing a way of health promotion by imitating five animals' action, namely tiger, bear, deer, ape, and bird. It was invented by Hua Tuo, the famous doctor in the Eastern Han Dynasty, on the basis of previous study. This collection is one of the five exercises—the tiger.

Preserved in National Library of China

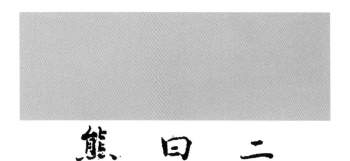

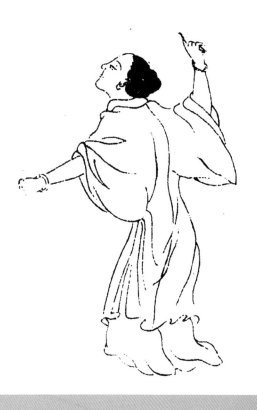

《五禽戏图谱·熊戏》

清

选自席裕康《内外功图说辑要》。此为五禽戏之二——熊戏。

中国国家图书馆藏

Wu Qin Xi Tu Pu-Bear Exercises

Qing Dynasty

The picture was selected from *Nei Wai Gong Tu Shuo Ji Yao* (Graphic Summary of Exercises to Benefit Inner Organs, Muscle and Bone) compiled by Xi Yukang. This collection is one of the five exercises—the bear.

Preserved in National Library of China

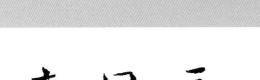

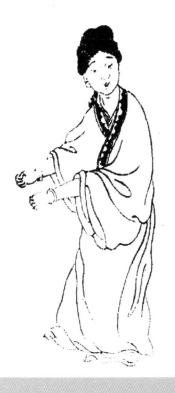

《五禽戏图谱·鹿戏》

清

选自席裕康《内外功图说辑要》。此为五禽
戏之三——鹿戏。

中国国家图书馆藏

Wu Qin Xi Tu Pu-Deer Exercises

Qing Dynasty

The picture was selected from *Nei Wai Gong Tu Shuo Ji Yao* (Graphic Summary of Exercises to Benefit Inner Organs, Muscle and Bone) compiled by Xi Yukang. This collection is one of the five exercises—the deer.

Preserved in National Library of China

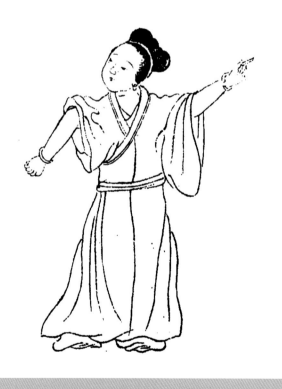

四 曰 猿

《五禽戏图谱·猿戏》

清

选自席裕康《内外功图说辑要》。此为五禽
戏之四——猿戏。

中国国家图书馆藏

Wu Qin Xi Tu Pu-Ape Exercises

Qing Dynasty

The picture was selected from *Nei Wai Gong Tu Shuo Ji Yao* (Graphic Summary of Exercises to Benefit Inner Organs, Muscle and Bone) compiled by Xi Yukang. This collection is one of the five exercises—the ape.

Preserved in National Library of China

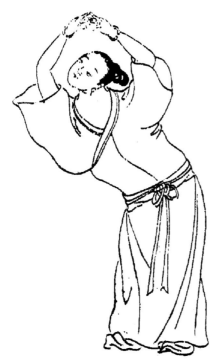

《五禽戏图谱·鸟戏》

清

选自席裕康《内外功图说辑要》。此为五禽戏之五——鸟戏。

中国国家图书馆藏

Wu Qin Xi Tu Pu-Bird Exercises

Qing Dynasty

The picture was selected from *Nei Wai Gong Tu Shuo Ji Yao* (Graphic Summary of Exercises to Benefit Inner Organs, Muscle and Bone) compiled by Xi Yukang. This collection is one of the five exercises—the bird.

Preserved in National Library of China

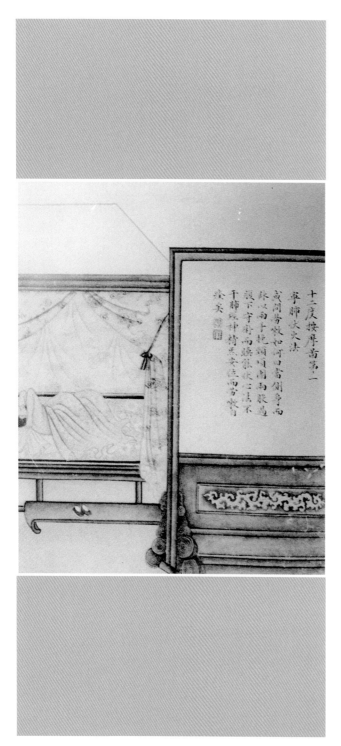

清人绘《十二度按摩图》之宁肺伏火法

清

该图谱系清朝人以按摩养生保健为载体绘制而成的。全谱共 12 幅，每幅图像生动逼真，并配有简明易懂的文字说明。从图谱的形式看，均属徒手按摩，是当时养生保健中按摩形式的重要形象依据。此为《十二度按摩图》之宁肺伏火法。

中国医史博物馆藏

Twelve Pictures of Massages in Qing Dynasty: " Ning Fei Fu Huo Fa"

Qing Dynasty

The twelve pictures were painted in the Qing Dynasty based on the theory of maintaining health through massage. Each of it is vivid and lively, with terse and perspicuous explanations. These twelve pictures of bare-handed massage are the important reference for massage methods in the Qing Dynasty. This collection is one of the pictures, depicting the massage that can reduce the pathogenic fire and tranquilize the lung (Ning Fei Fu Huo Fa).

Preserved in Chinese Medical History Museum

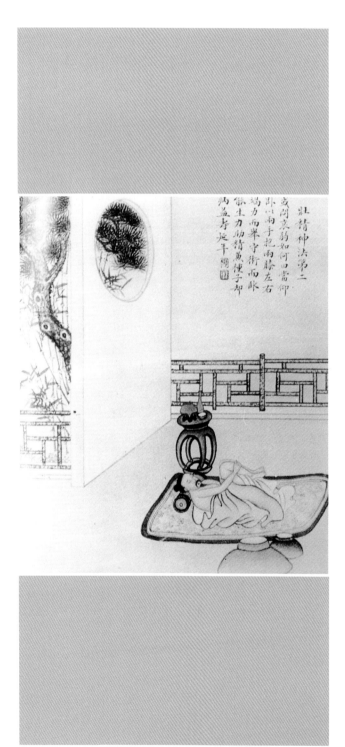

清人绘《十二度按摩图》之壮精神法

清

该图谱系清朝人以按摩养生保健为载体绘制而成的。此为《十二度按摩图》之壮精神法。

中国医史博物馆藏

Twelve Pictures of Massages in Qing Dynasty: "Zhuang Jing Shen Fa"

Qing Dynasty

The twelve pictures were painted in the Qing Dynasty based on the theory of maintaining health through massage. This is one of them, depicting the massage for refreshment (Zhuang Jing Shen Fa).

Preserved in Chinese Medical History Museum

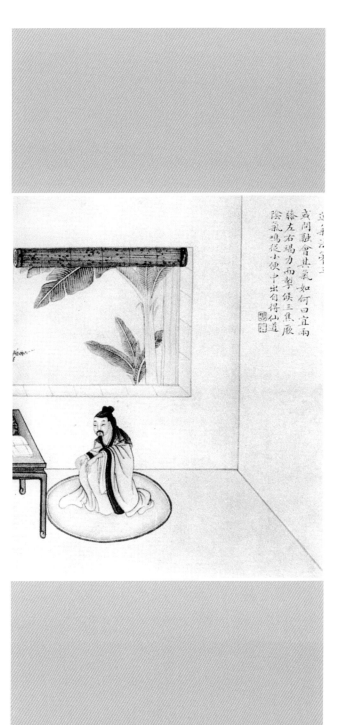

清人绘《十二度按摩图》之运气法

清

该图谱系清朝人以按摩养生保健为载体绘制而成的。此为《十二度按摩图》之运气法。

中国医史博物馆藏

Twelve Pictures of Massages in Qing Dynasty: "Yun Qi Fa"

Qing Dynasty

The twelve pictures were painted in the Qing Dynasty based on the theory of maintaining health through massage. This is one of them, depicting the massage to conduct Qi (Yun Qi Fa). Preserved in Chinese Medical History Museum

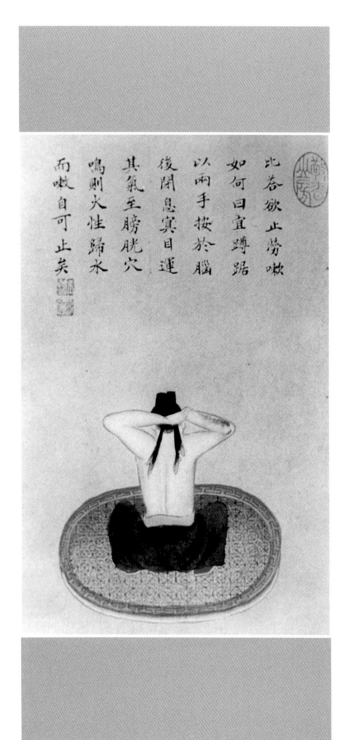

此若欲止劳嗽
如何曰宜蹲踞
以两手按於脑
後開息閉目運
其氣至膀胱穴
嗚則火性歸水
而嗽自可止矣

《导引图》之止痨嗽导引式

清

《导引图》为清代工笔彩绘，共绘有养生和治疗各种疾病的导引、按摩术式 24 种，每幅图像生动逼真，并配有简明易懂的文字说明。此为《导引图》术式之止痨嗽导引式。

中国中医科学院图书馆藏

Guidance Pictures: Relieving Cough

Qing Dynasty

These colored *Guidance Pictures*, characterized by fine brushwork, recorded 24 kinds of massage methods and guidance for maintaining health and treating various diseases. Each picture is vivid and lively, with terse and perspicuous explanations. As one page of them, this picture depicts the method of relieving cough caused by tuberculosis.

Preserved in Library of China Academy of Chinese Medical Sciences

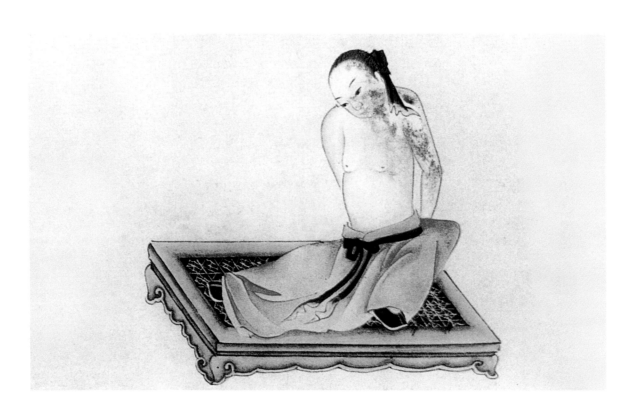

《导引图》之练元精按摩式

清

此为《导引图》中按摩术式之练元精按摩式。

中国中医科学院图书馆藏

Guidance Pictures: Promoting the Primordial Essence

Qing Dynasty

As one page of the *Guidance Pictures*, this picture depicts the massage method of promoting the primordial essence.

Preserved in Library of China Academy of Chinese Medical Sciences

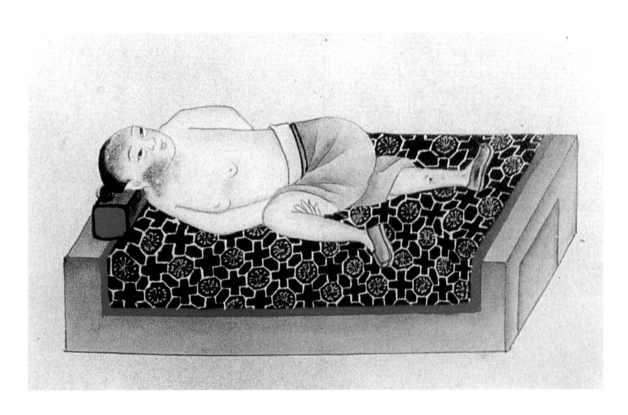

《导引图》之养元真按摩式

清

此为《导引图》中按摩术式之养元真按摩式。

中国中医科学院图书馆藏

Guidance Pictures: Recuperating the Primordial Essence

Qing Dynasty

As one page of the *Guidance Pictures*, this picture depicts the massage method of recuperating the primordial

essence.

Preserved in Library of China Academy of Chinese Medical Sciences

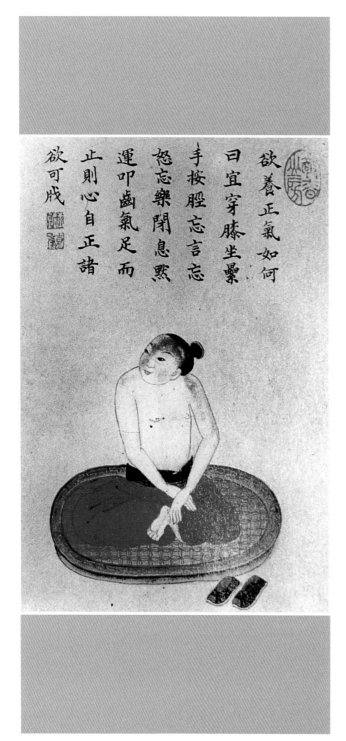

欲養正氣如何
曰宜穿膝坐壘
手按脛忘言忘
怒忘樂閉息然
運叩齒氣足而
止則心自正諸
欲可戒

《导引图》之养正气导引式

清

此为《导引图》中按摩术式之养正气导引式。

中国中医科学院图书馆藏

Guidance Pictures: Recuperating the Vital Energy

Qing Dynasty

As one page of the *Guidance Pictures*, this picture depicts the massage method of recuperating the vital energy.

Preserved in Library of China Academy of Chinese Medical Sciences

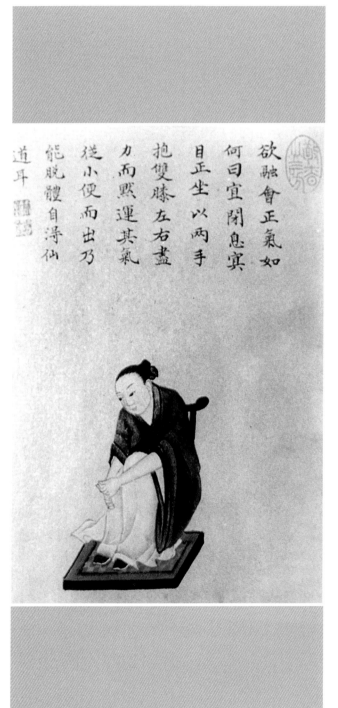

欲融會正氣如
何日宜閉息宴
目正坐以兩手
抱雙膝左右盡
力而黙運其氣
從小便而出乃
能脫體自得仙
道耳

《导引图》之融合正气导引式

清

此为《导引图》中按摩术式之融合正气导引式。

中国中医科学院图书馆藏

Guidance Pictures: Fusing the Vital Energy

Qing Dynasty

As one page of the *Guidance Pictures*, this picture depicts the massage method of fusing the vital energy.

Preserved in Library of China Academy of Chinese Medical Sciences

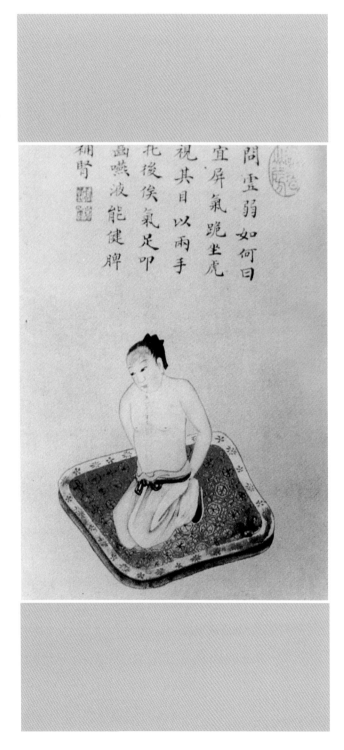

問靈翁如何日
宜屏氣跪坐虎
視其目以兩手
托後俟氣足叩
齒嗾液能健脾
補腎

《导引图》之补虚导引式

清

此为《导引图》中按摩术式之补虚导引式。

中国中医科学院图书馆藏

Guidance Pictures: Tonifying the Deficiency

Qing Dynasty

As one page of the *Guidance Pictures*, this picture depicts the massage method of tonifying the deficiency.

Preserved in Library of China Academy of Chinese Medical Sciences

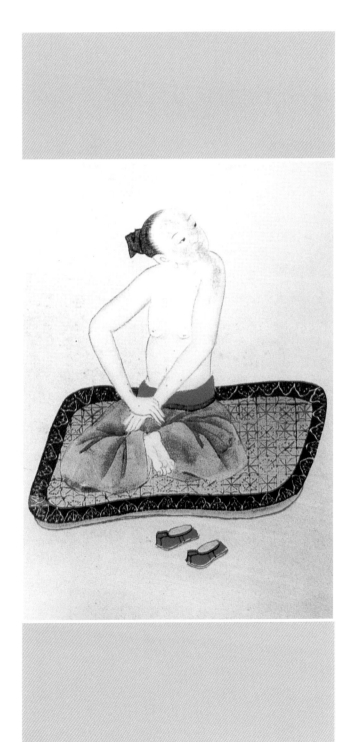

《导引图》之治遗精按摩式

清

此为《导引图》中按摩术式之治遗精按摩式。

中国中医科学院图书馆藏

Guidance Pictures: Treating Spermatorrhea

Qing Dynasty

As one page of the *Guidance Pictures*, this picture depicts the massage method of treating spermatorrhea.

Preserved in Library of China Academy of Chinese Medical Sciences

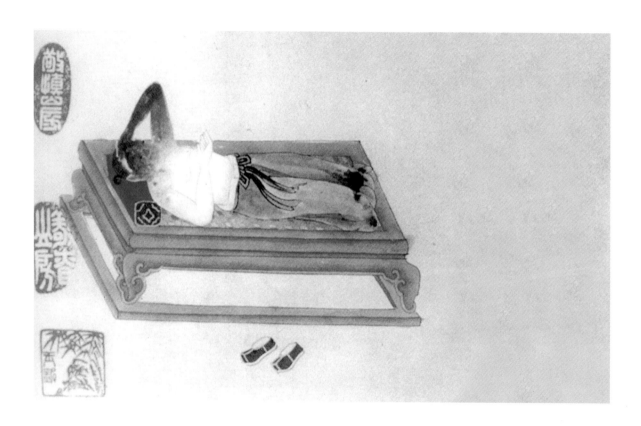

《导引图》之补气血按摩式

清

此为《导引图》中按摩术式之补气血按摩式。

中国中医科学院图书馆藏

Guidance Pictures: Tonifying Qi-blood

Qing Dynasty

As one page of the *Guidance Pictures*, this picture depicts the massage method of tonifying Qi-blood.

Preserved in Library of China Academy of Chinese Medical Sciences

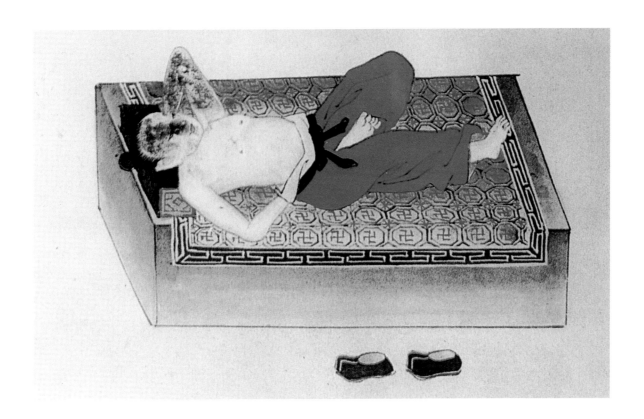

《导引图》之治元气虚按摩式

清

此为《导引图》中按摩术式之治元气虚按摩式。

中国中医科学院图书馆藏

Guidance Pictures: Tonifying the Deficiency of Vital Energy

Qing Dynasty

As one page of the *Guidance Pictures*, this picture depicts the massage method of tonifying the deficiency of vital energy.

Preserved in Library of China Academy of Chinese Medical Sciences

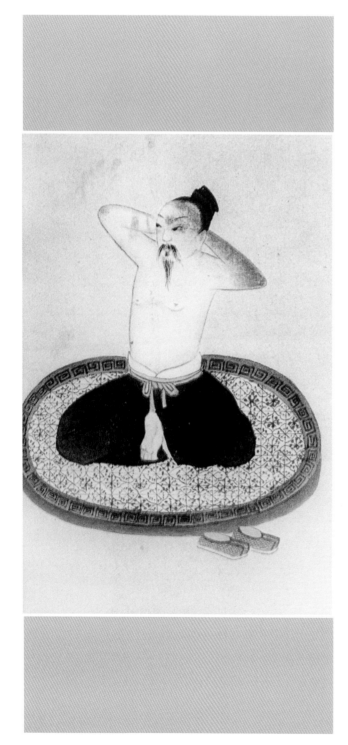

《导引图》之治眩晕按摩式

清

此为《导引图》中按摩术式之治眩晕按摩式。

中国中医科学院图书馆藏

Guidance Pictures: Treating Dizziness

Qing Dynasty

As one page of the *Guidance Pictures*, this picture depicts the massage method of treating dizziness.

Preserved in Library of China Academy of Chinese Medical Sciences

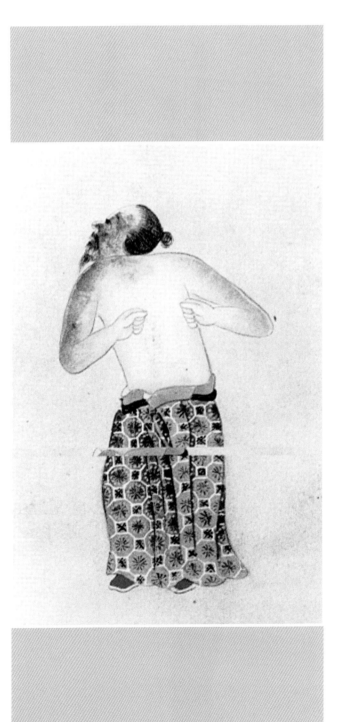

《导引图》之理瘀血按摩式

清

此为《导引图》中按摩术式之理瘀血按摩式。

中国中医科学院图书馆藏

Guidance Pictures: Cleaning Stagnate

Qing Dynasty

As one page of the *Guidance Pictures*, this picture depicts the massage method of cleaning stagnate.

Preserved in Library of China Academy of Chinese Medical Sciences

為長力延年之一助云爾
坦夫自新氏錄
峕在
道光重光赤奮若病月望日
後學王俊謹書

調氣煉外丹圖
凡行此功者須擇潔淨處面向東
立舌舐上腭調其氣息任其出入
首微仰目微上視通身不可用力
一有用力則氣不貫至手拳矣每
行一式須默數七七四十九字畢
即接行下式不可間斷斷則氣散

第一套第一式
面向東立首微仰目微上視兩足
與肩齊腳跕平不可前後參差兩
臂垂下肘微曲兩掌下十指朝前
默數七七四十九字每數一字十
指想拄上蹻兩掌想拄下搽穀四
十九字即四十九蹻搽也

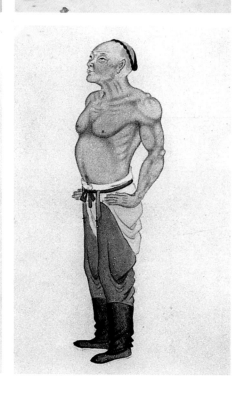

清人绘《调气练外丹图式》书影

清

练功图谱。所载功法 3 套，简便易行，图文并
茂。此为其中 4 幅书影。

中国医史博物馆藏

Book Photograph of *Tiao Qi Lian Wai Dan Tu Shi*

Qing Dynasty

Tiao Qi Lian Wai Dan Tu Shi (Figure of Regulating Breathing and External Alchemy) recorded 3 sets of Qigong arts with both pictures and explanations, which is convenient and practical. These are four pages from it.

Preserved in Chinese Medical History Museum

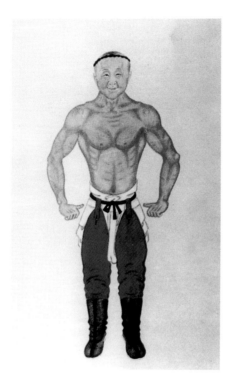

即四十九緊與蹺也　大指蹺一蹺數四十九字　身每數一字拳加一緊兩　為拳掌背向前兩大指朝　前式數字畢即將八指叠　第二式

清人绘《调气练外丹图式》第一套第二式

清

左下图为第一套第二式文字说明。

中国医史博物馆藏

Tiao Qi Lian Wai Dan Tu Shi (Second Posture, First Set)

Qing Dynasty

On the lower left of the picture is the explanation for the second posture in the first set of *Tiao Qi Lian Wai Dan Tu Shi* (Figure of Regulating Breathing and External Alchemy).

Preserved in Chinese Medical History Museum

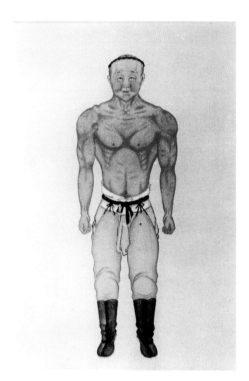

拳加一緊　伸矣虎口朝前每數一字　下一搋肘之微曲者至此　中指中節上為拳趁勢往　前式數字畢將大指叠在　第三式

清人绘《调气练外丹图式》第一套第三式

清

左下图为第一套第三式文字说明。

中国医史博物馆藏

Tiao Qi Lian Wai Dan Tu Shi (Third Posture, First Set)

Qing Dynasty

On the lower left of the picture is the explanation for the third posture in the first set of *Tiao Qi Lian Wai Dan Tu Shi* (Figure of Regulating Breathing and External Alchemy).

Preserved in Chinese Medical History Museum

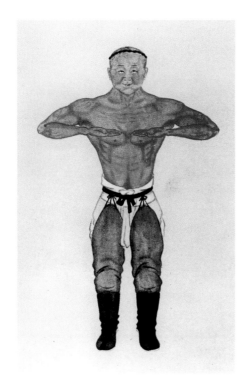

指字上伸寸字天
尖想寸黙想接末
手许數手頭許
心十四心叁闲
黳九十黳呑人
平字字翻氣書
想每每向三
氣一一上口
貫十端畢
十接二盉將
頭三乳拳

清人绘《调气练外丹图式》第二
套第一式

清

左下图为第二套第一式文字说明。

中国医史博物馆藏

Tiao Qi Lian Wai Dan Tu Shi (First
Posture, Second Set)

Qing Dynasty

On the lower left of the picture is the explanation
for the first posture in the second set of *Tiao
Qi Lian Wai Dan Tu Shi* (Figure of Regulating
Breathing and External Alchemy).

Preserved in Chinese Medical History Museum

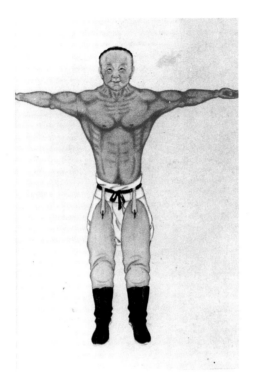

清人绘《调气练外丹图式》第二套第二式

清

左下图为第二套第二式文字说明。

中国医史博物馆藏

Tiao Qi Lian Wai Dan Tu Shi (Second Posture, Second Set)

Qing Dynasty

On the lower left of the picture is the explanation for the second posture in the second set of *Tiao Qi Lian Wai Dan Tu Shi* (Figure of Regulating Breathing and External Alchemy).

Preserved in Chinese Medical History Museum

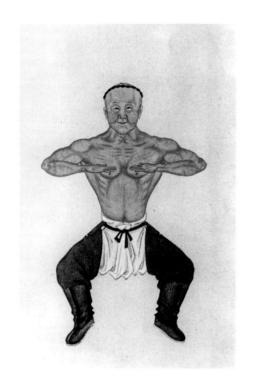

清人绘《调气练外丹图式》第三套第一式

清

左下图为第三套第一式文字说明。

中国医史博物馆藏

Tiao Qi Lian Wai Dan Tu Shi (First Posture, Third Set)

Qing Dynasty

On the lower left of the picture is the explanation for the first posture in the third set of *Tiao Qi Lian Wai Dan Tu Shi* (Figure of Regulating Breathing and External Alchemy).

Preserved in Chinese Medical History Museum

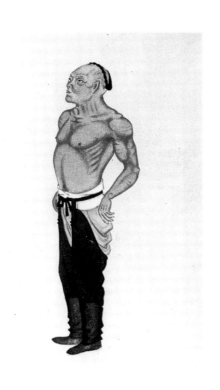

清人绘《调气练外丹图式》第三套第五式

清

左下图为第三套第五式文字说明。

中国医史博物馆藏

Tiao Qi Lian Wai Dan Tu Shi (Fifth Posture, Third Set)

Qing Dynasty

On the lower left of the picture is the explanation for the fifth posture in the third set of *Tiao Qi Lian Wai Dan Tu Shi* (Figure of Regulating Breathing and External Alchemy).

Preserved in Chinese Medical History Museum

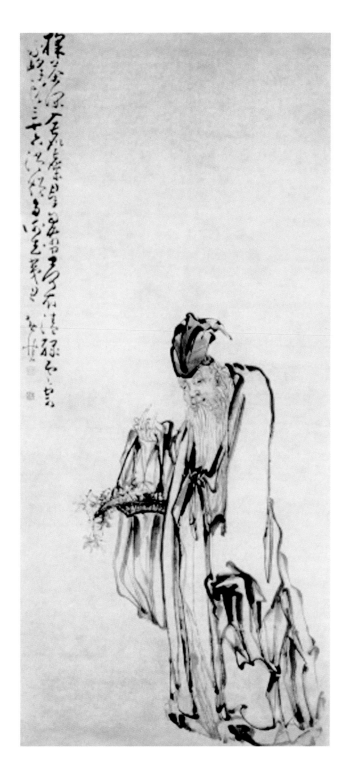

采茶老翁图轴

清

纵 137 厘米，横 64.5 厘米

淡设色写意。图中画一白髯老者，青巾布衣，
手提茶篮，款款独行，似自山中采茶归来。
形象生动准确，用笔豪劲纵逸，设色淡雅。
左上题七言绝句，自署"黄慎"，下钤两方
印记，文为"瘿瓢""黄慎"。

烟台市博物馆藏

Painting Scroll of Tea-picking Old Man

Qing Dynasty

Vertical Length 137 cm/ Horizontal Length 64.5 cm

In this free-sketch painting, a white-bearded old man in black hat and cotton garment is walking alone leisurely carrying a tea basket. It seems he is coming back after picking tea leaves in the mountains. The painting has an accurate and vivid image and is drawn in strong and unconstrained style with light color. A seven-character quatrain is inscribed on the upper left of the painting. Under the signature "Huang Shen" are two seals reading "Ying Piao" and "Huang Shen".

Preserved in Yantai Museum

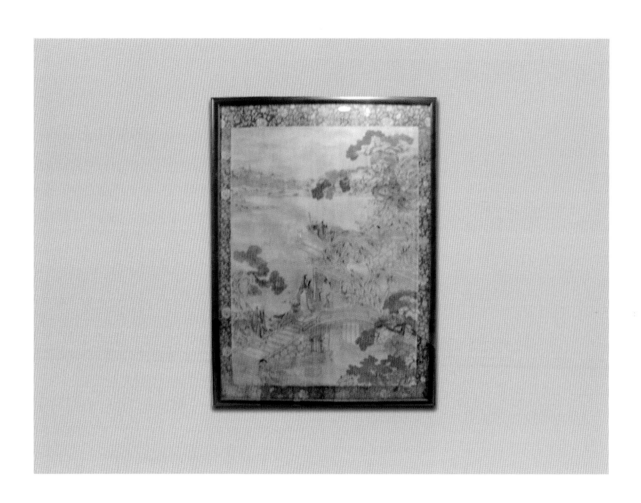

缂丝画

清

宽 80 厘米，高 116 厘米

此图表达了人们为寿星祝寿的场景和愿望，由四川文物拍卖公司征集。

成都中医药大学中医药传统文化博物馆藏

Ke Si Painting

Qing Dynasty

Width 80 cm/ Height 116 cm

The painting describes the situation of people congratulating an elderly person on his birthday. It was collected from Sichuan Cultural Relics Auction Company.

Preserved in Museum of Traditional Chinese Medicine Culture, Chengdu University of Traditional Chinese Medicine

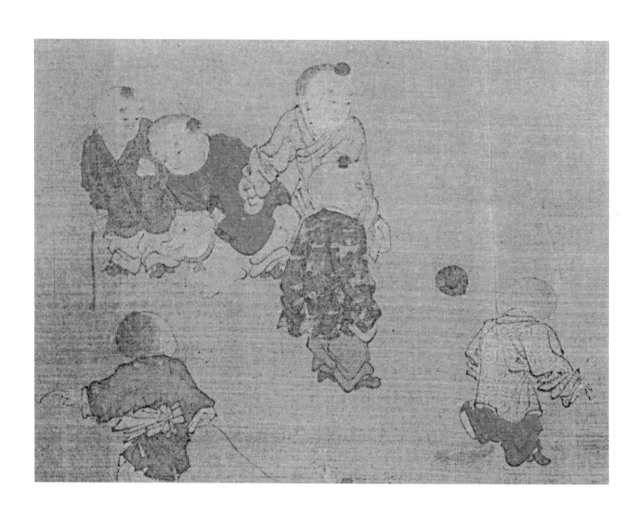

佚名《蹴鞠图》册页

清

纵 30 厘米，横 35 厘米

画面描绘的是一组童戏图案，右边有三个儿童正在玩蹴鞠，中间一球已经被踢起。左边有三位儿童正在嬉戏观看。

中国体育博物馆藏

Album of *Cu Ju Tu* (Anonymous)

Qing Dynasty

Vertical Length 30 cm/ Horizontal Length 35 cm

The painting described the situation of children playing the game of Cuju, a kind of ancient football. On the right are three children playing Cuju. On the left are three children playing and watching.

Preserved in China Sports Museum

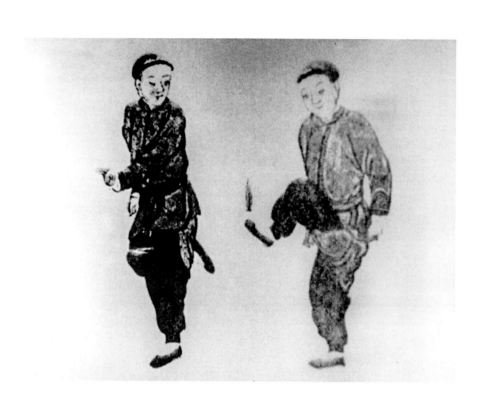

踢毽子风俗画

清

此图收于中国国家图书馆藏的《北京民间风俗百图》中，画面展示了清代北京人在闲暇时节踢毽子游戏的情景。

中国国家图书馆藏

Folk Painting of Kicking Shuttlecock

Qing Dynasty

The painting was included in *Bei Jing Min Jian Feng Su Bai Tu* (the collection of the paintings of folk artists in the Qing Dynasty) preserved in National Library of China. It depicted the situation of people in Beijing kicking shuttlecock in their leisure time in the Qing Dynasty.

Preserved in National Library of China

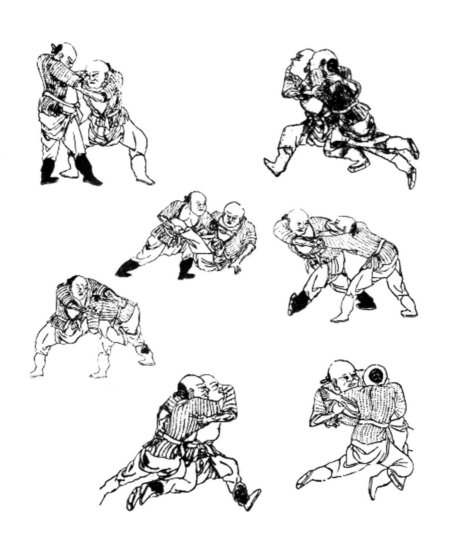

木刻《摔跤图》拓本

清

长 15.5~24.5 厘米，宽 13.4~18.2 厘米，厚 1.3~9 厘米

木制版刻。图中的两位摔跤手，皆脑后梳有鬐辫，身着短衣搭链，腰束宽带。一人着黑靴，另一人着白靴。木刻摔跤图上动作姿态不一，但具有连续性，应为一摔跤连续动作的范本。

故宫博物院藏

Woodcut *Painting of Wrestling* (Rubbing)

Qing Dynasty

Length 15.5–24.5 cm/ Width 13.4–18.2 cm/ Thickness 1.3–9 cm

This set of wrestling paintings is woodcut edition. The two wrestlers in the painting are both in short jackets and loose girdles with a bun or braid overhead. One is in black boots and the other in white ones. Though the paintings have different images in action and posture, they are consecutive and can form a model of continuous wrestling actions.

Preserved in The Palace Museum

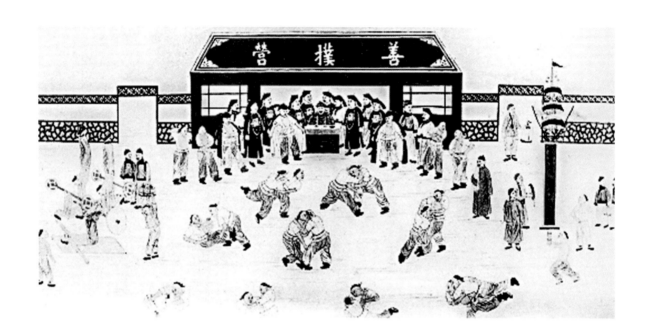

《善扑营摔跤图》

清

善扑营是清代特设的一类专门挑选八旗勇士演练摔跤、射箭和驯马技艺的习武机构。此图即是以善扑营的摔跤为主题绘制而成的，画面描绘了皇帝在大臣们的陪同下，例行巡幸善扑营观看摔跤手们摔跤的情形。

故宫博物院藏

Painting of Wrestling in Shan Pu Ying

Qing Dynasty

Shan Pu Ying is a Wushu practice institution in the Qing Dynasty specially set to select the warriors from the "Eight Banners (the military establishment of Manchu in the Qing Dynasty)" for practicing wrestling, archery and taming horses. The theme of this painting is the wrestling in Shan Pu Ying. It depicted that the emperor, accompanied by the principal officials, was doing the routine inspection in Shan Pu Ying and watching the wrestling.

Preserved in The Palace Museum

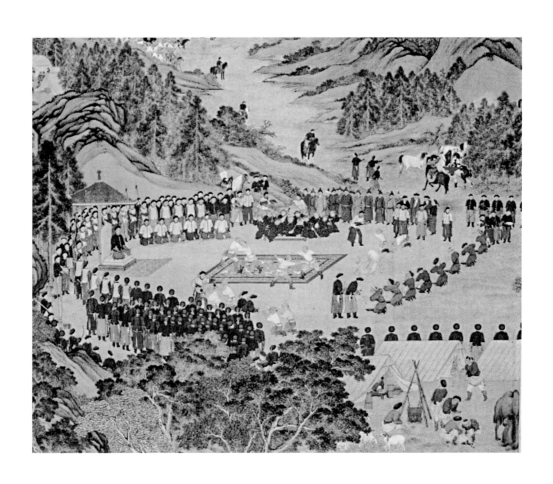

《塞宴四事图》轴局部

清

原图：纵 320 厘米，横 560 厘米

《塞宴四事图》轴记录了乾隆皇帝在承德避暑山庄大宴群臣时的盛况。本画面选录的是其中描写摔跤活动时的一个场面，中间地毯上两对光着头、穿白色对襟搭链的摔跤手，正在进行"布库"（类似今天的中国式摔跤）比赛；地毯右边地上的一对摔跤手，则赤膊光脚，正在进行"厄鲁持"（类似今天国际上的古典式摔跤）比赛。此图是清代摔跤活动的真实写照。

故宫博物院藏

Scroll Painting of *Sai Yan Si Shi Tu* (Partial)

Qing Dynasty

Original Painting: Vertical Length 320 cm/ Horizontal Length 560 cm

The painting *Sai Yan Si Shi Tu* recorded the grand occasion of Emperor Qianlong entertaining the officials in Chengde Imperial Summer Resort. This part depicted the wrestling activity at that time. In the middle of the carpet, two bald wrestlers in white jackets with buttons down the front are playing "Buccoo" (an activity which seems like the Chinese wrestling nowadays). Right beside the carpet, two barebacked and barefoot wrestlers are playing "Olot" (an activity which seems like the international Greco-Roman wrestling nowadays). The part of the painting is a real reflection of wrestling activity in the Qing Dynasty.

Preserved in The Palace Museum

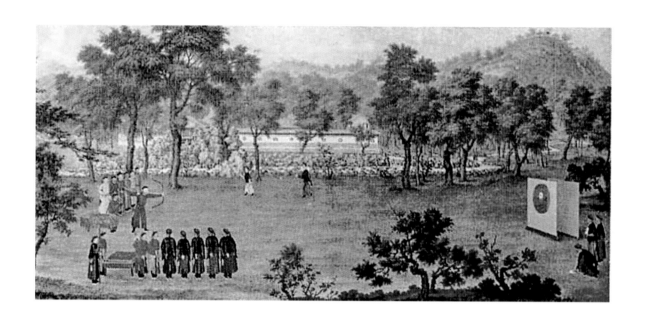

（法）王致诚《乾隆射箭油画挂屏》

清

纵 105.3 厘米，横 224.1 厘米

此画以清高宗乾隆皇帝在避暑山庄射箭习武为题材绘成。图中乾隆皇帝在大臣们的陪同下，正在执弓射靶。

故宫博物院藏

Qian Long She Jian You Hua Gua Ping by Wang Zhicheng (France)

Qing Dynasty

Vertical Length 105.3 cm / Horizontal Length 224.1 cm

The theme of the oil painting is about the Emperor Qianlong shooting and practicing Martial Arts in Chengde Imperial Summer Resort. In the painting, accompanied by officials, Emperor Qianlong is holding the bow and shooting.

Preserved in The Palace Museum

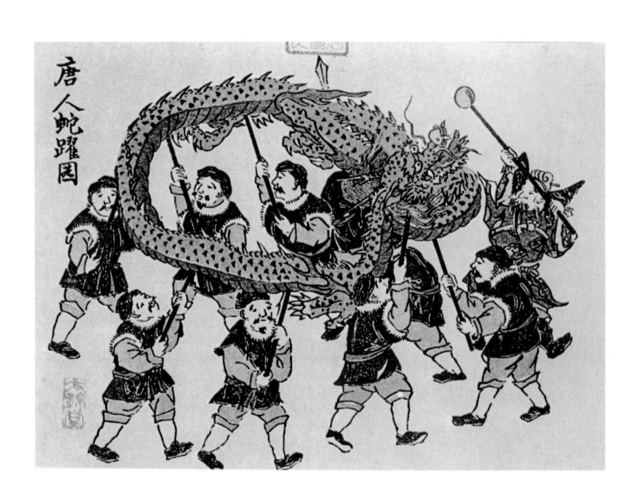

舞龙图年画

清

画面印有"太锦堂"三字，当为"太锦堂"年画作品。图中八位艺人同执一巨龙在舞弄，所舞之龙已盘成圆圈状，龙首有一艺人在作导引。

日本长崎市立博物馆藏

New Year Picture of Dragon Dance

Qing Dynasty

In this new year picture, there are three characters reading "Tai Jin Tang", which is the name of its producer. In the picture, eight dancers are holding the dragon and waving it to form a circle. A dancer is leading in front of the dragon.

Preserved in Nagasaki Museum of Japan

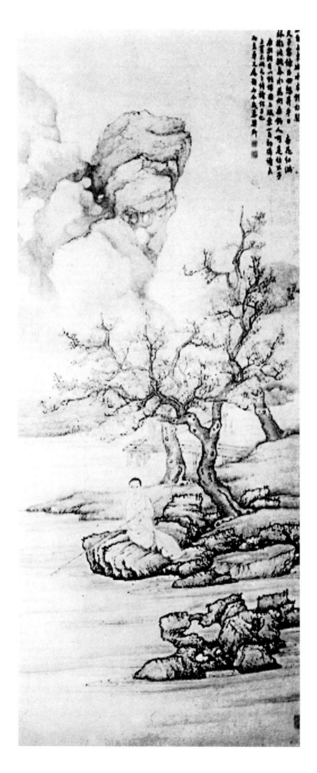

禹之鼎《丙炎杏溪垂钓图》轴

清

图中背景为山石、柏树衬托下的溪水，水面上架一竹木小桥。枯树下面的溪水边，一身穿长袍的垂钓者正执竿而钓。画面表现了一种安逸、静谧的垂钓气氛。

故宫博物院藏

Scroll Painting of *Bing Yan Xing Xi Chui Diao Tu* by Yu Zhiding

Qing Dynasty

The background of the painting is a stream set off by the mountains, rocks and cypresses. Over the stream is a bridge made of bamboo and wood. By the side of the stream under a dry tree, a fisher in long gown is holding the rod and fishing. The painting is in a comfortable and quiet atmosphere.

Preserved in The Palace Museum

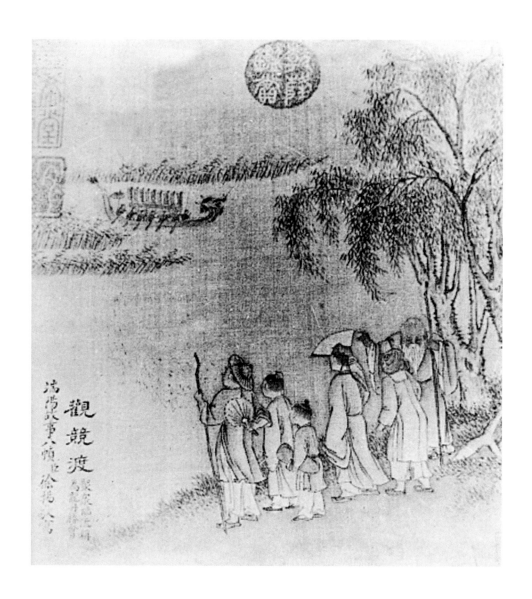

徐场《观竞渡》

清

这是画家以端午之故事绘制而成的一幅争相观看龙舟竞渡情景的画卷，图中行于水上的龙舟、划舟的人物以及岸边的观看者被描绘的生动精巧，充满情趣。

故宫博物院藏

Painting of *Watching Dragon Boat Racing* by Xu Chang

Qing Dynasty

Based on the story of Dragon Boat Festival, the painting describes the scene of people eagerly watching dragon boat racing. In the painting, the dragon boats in the river, the people rowing the boats and the people watching on the bank are all depicted vividly and ingeniously. It was full of fun.

Preserved in The Palace Museum

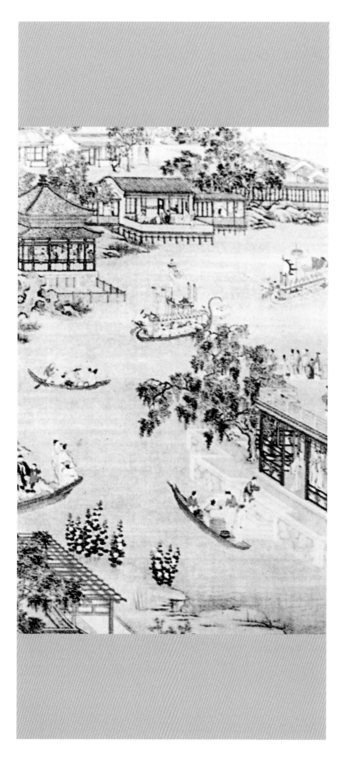

《十二月令图》局部

清

这里选取的是由清代画院绘制的《十二月令图》中一幅描述龙舟竞渡活动的画面。图中表现了五月端午节期间，身着不同服装的桨手们，在鼓声震震中奋力划水、竞舟并进的情景。

故宫博物院藏

Painting of *Shi Er Yue Ling Tu* (Partial)

Qing Dynasty

The part selected here is a scene of the painting *Shi Er Yue Ling Tu* (a painting of the scenes in twelve months) drawn by Imperial Art Academy in the Qing Dynasty, depicting the scene of dragon boat racing. It shows that on the Dragon Boat Festival in May, the boatmen in different costumes struggle to paddle and race in the sound of drums.

Preserved in The Palace Museum

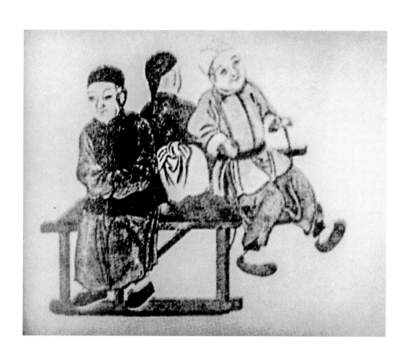

拉冰床风俗画

清

选自《北京民间风俗百图》，画面展示了清代的北京人在结冰后的护城河上做拉冰床游戏的情景。这种床以木做成，下安铁条两根，每当人们进行冰嬉活动时，便以绳拉之，在冰上滑行，别有一番情趣。

中国国家图书馆藏

Folk Painting of Pulling Sledge

Qing Dynasty

Selected from *Bei Jing Min Jian Feng Su Bai Tu* (the collection of the paintings of folk artists), the painting depicts the scene in which in the Qing Dynasty, people in Beijing played the game of pulling sledge on the frozen city moat. This kind of sledge was made of wood with two iron rods at the bottom. When people did ice activities, they pulled the sledge by ropes and made it slide on the ice. It was of much fun.

Preserved in National Library of China

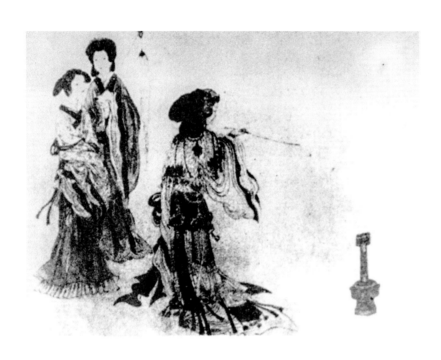

任熊《玉女投壶图》

清

图中绘有一位玉女在执箭投壶，旁有两个侍女观看。画面中投壶之壶为明清流行之典型样式。

故宫博物院藏

Painting of *Yu Nü Tou Hu Tu* by Ren Xiong

Qing Dynasty

The painting depicts the scene in which a teenage girl is holding arrows and throwing them into a pot. Two maids are watching by the side. The pot in the painting was in the popular style in the Ming and Qing Dynasties.

Preserved in The Palace Museum

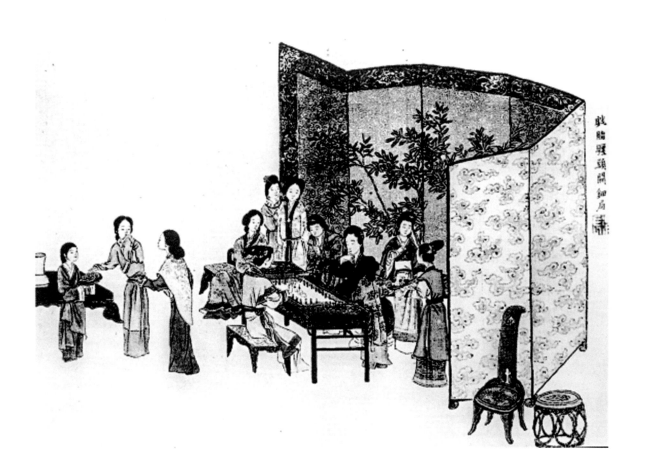

任熊《双陆图》

清

图中两贵妇正专注地在双陆局边对弈，旁边有观棋的仕女，也有奉盘的侍女。整个画面生动活泼，显示了内室女眷打双陆的场景。

故宫博物院藏

Painting of *Shuang Lu Tu* (Playing Backgammon) by Ren Xiong

Qing Dynasty

In the painting, two ladies are concentrating on playing backgammon. There are ladies watching by the side and maids holding dishes. The whole painting is vivid and lively, depicting the situation of family women playing backgammon.

Preserved in The Palace Museum

索 引

（馆藏地按拼音字母排序）

Index

450

Chinese Medical Association/ Museum of Chinese Medicine, Shanghai University of Traditional Chinese Medicine

参考文献

[1] 李经纬.中国古代医史图录 [M].北京：人民卫生出版社，1992.

[2] 傅维康，李经纬，林昭庚.中国医学通史：文物图谱卷 [M].北京：人民卫生出版社，2000.

[3] 和中浚，吴鸿洲.中华医学文物图集 [M].成都：四川人民出版社，2001.

[4] 上海中医药博物馆.上海中医药博物馆馆藏珍品 [M].上海：上海科学技术出版社，2013.

[5] 西藏自治区博物馆.西藏博物馆 [M].北京：五洲传播出版社，2005.

[6] 崔乐泉.中国古代体育文物图录：中英文本 [M].北京：中华书局，2000.

[7] 张金明，陆雪春.中国古铜镜鉴赏图录 [M].北京：中国民族摄影艺术出版社，2002.

[8] 文物精华编辑委员会.文物精华 [M].北京：文物出版社，1964.

[9] 谭维四.湖北出土文物精华 [M].武汉：湖北教育出版社，2001.

[10] 常州市博物馆.常州文物精华 [M].北京：文物出版社，1998.

[11] 镇江博物馆.镇江文物精华 [M].合肥：黄山书社，1997.

[12] 贵州省文化厅，贵州省博物馆.贵州文物精华 [M].贵阳：贵州人民出版社，2005.

[13] 徐良玉.扬州馆藏文物精华 [M].南京：江苏古籍出版社，2001.

[14] 昭陵博物馆，陕西历史博物馆.昭陵文物精华 [M].西安：陕西人民美术出版社，1991.

[15] 南通博物苑.南通博物苑文物精华 [M].北京：文物出版社，2005.

[16] 邯郸市文物研究所.邯郸文物精华 [M].北京：文物出版社，2005.

[17] 张秀生，刘友恒，聂连顺，等.中国河北正定文物精华 [M].北京：文化艺术出版社，1998.

[18] 陕西省咸阳市文物局.咸阳文物精华 [M].北京：文物出版社，2002.

[19] 安阳市文物管理局.安阳文物精华 [M].北京：文物出版社，2004.

[20] 深圳市博物馆.深圳市博物馆文物精华 [M].北京：文物出版社，1998.

[21]《中国文物精华》编辑委员会.中国文物精华（1993）[M].北京：文物出版社，1993.

[22] 夏路，刘永生 . 山西省博物馆馆藏文物精华 [M]. 太原：山西人民出版社，1999.

[23] 文物精华编辑委员会 . 文物精华 [M]. 北京：文物出版社，1957.

[24] 山西博物院，湖北省博物馆 . 荆楚长歌：九连墩楚墓出土文物精华 [M]. 太原：山西人民出版社，2011.

[25] 刘广堂，石金鸣，宋建忠 . 晋国雄风：山西出土两周文物精华 [M]. 沈阳：万卷出版公司，2009.

[26] 沈君山，王国平，单迎红 . 滦平博物馆馆藏文物精华 [M]. 北京：中国文联出版社，2012.

[27] 张家口市博物馆 . 张家口市博物馆馆藏文物精华 [M]. 北京：科学出版社，2011.

[28] 浙江省文物考古研究所 . 浙江考古精华 [M]. 北京：文物出版社，1999.

[29] 故宫博物院 . 故宫雕刻珍萃 [M]. 北京：紫禁城出版社，2004.

[30] 故宫博物院紫禁城出版社 . 故宫博物院藏宝录 [M]. 上海：上海文艺出版社，1986.

[31] 首都博物馆 . 大元三都 [M]. 北京：科学出版社，2016.

[32] 新疆维吾尔自治区博物馆 . 新疆出土文物 [M]. 北京：文物出版社，1975.

[33] 王兴伊，段逸山 . 新疆出土涉医文书辑校 [M]. 上海：上海科学技术出版社，2016.

[34] 刘学春 . 刍议医药卫生文物的概念与分类标准 [J]. 中华中医药杂志，2016，31（11）:4406-4409.

[35] 上海古籍出版社 . 中国艺海 [M]. 上海：上海古籍出版社，1994.

[36] 紫都，岳鑫 . 一生必知的 200 件国宝 [M]. 呼和浩特：远方出版社，2005.

[37] 谭维四 . 湖北出土文物精华 [M]. 武汉：湖北教育出版社，2001.

[38] 张建青 . 青海彩陶收藏与鉴赏 [M]. 北京：中国文史出版社，2007.

[39] 银景琦 . 仡佬族文物 [M]. 南宁：广西人民出版社，2014.

[40] 廖果，梁峻，李经纬 . 东西方医学的反思与前瞻 [M]. 北京：中医古籍出版社，2002.

[41] 梁峻，张志斌，廖果，等 . 中华医药文明史集论 [M]. 北京：中医古籍出版社，2003.

[42] 郑蓉，庄乾竹，刘聪，等 . 中国医药文化遗产考论 [M]. 北京：中医古籍出版社，2005.